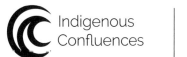

Indigenous
Confluences

MW01031599

Charlo

and Coll Thrush, *Series Editors*

INDIAN BLOOD

HIV and Colonial Trauma in
San Francisco's Two-Spirit Community

ANDREW J. JOLIVETTE

UNIVERSITY OF WASHINGTON PRESS

Seattle and London

Printed and bound in the United States of America
Typeset in Charter, a typeface designed by Matthew Carter
20 19 18 17 16   5 4 3 2 1

Portions of chapters 1 and 2 were previously published in Andrew Jolivette, "Indian Blood:
Two-Spirit Cultural Dissolution, Mixed-Race Identity, and Sexuality—A Journey of Return,"
in *Sociologists in Action: Race, Class, Gender, Sexuality*, ed. Kathleen Korgen, Jonathan
White, and Shelly White (Thousand Oaks, CA: Sage, 2014), 118–23, and in Andrew Jolivette,
"Indian Blood: HIV and Colonial Trauma in San Francisco's Two-Spirit Community," *HIV
Australia* 13, no. 3 (December 2015). Portions of chapter 1 were previously published in
Andrew Jolivette, "Two-Spirit Cultural Dissolution: HIV and Healing among Mixed-Race
American Indians," in *Mixed 3.0: Risk and Reward in the Digital Age*, ed. Ulli Ryder and
Marcia Dawkins (Los Angeles: USC Annenberg Press, 2015).

UNIVERSITY OF WASHINGTON PRESS
www.washington.edu/uwpress

LIBRARY OF CONGRESS CATALOGING-IN-PUBLICATION DATA
Names: Jolivette, Andrew, 1975–
Title: Indian blood : HIV and colonial trauma in San Francisco's two-spirit community /
    Andrew J. Jolivette.
Description: Seattle : University of Washington Press, 2016. | Includes bibliographical
    references and index.
Identifiers: LCCN 2015047434| ISBN 9780295998077 (hardcover : acid-free paper) |
    ISBN 9780295998503 (paperback : acid-free paper)
Subjects: LCSH: Two-spirit people—California—San Francisco—Social conditions.
    | Indian gays—California—San Francisco—Social conditions. | Racially mixed
    people—California—San Francisco—Social conditions. | Racially mixed people—
    California—San Francisco—Ethnic identity. | HIV-positive gay men—California—San
    Francisco—Social conditions. | Public health—California—San Francisco. | Indians
    of North America—Colonization—Social aspects. | Psychic trauma—Social aspects—
    United States. | Intergenerational relations—United States. | San Francisco (Calif.)—
    Ethnic relations.
Classification: LCC E98.S48 J65 2016 | DDC 305.8009794/61—dc23
LC record available at http://lccn.loc.gov/2015047434

In loving memory of my beautiful mother,
Annetta Donan Foster-Jolivette,
January 16, 1944–September 5, 2012

My first and best teacher . . .
Your lifeblood continues to nourish me and give me hope
and inspiration for a better and more just world

CONTENTS

PREFACE

Burning sage fills the room at the Native American AIDS Project in San Francisco with pungent smoke. It's a cold winter day when I begin my first focus group with gay, Two-Spirit, and transgender American Indians who also identify as mixed-race. As each participant enters the room, I introduce myself and explain that the goal of this project is to understand how we can reduce rates of HIV/AIDS infection in American Indian and Indigenous communities. I also suggest that this is a story about healing, not about sickness. This is, I tell them, a story that will produce meaningful interventions for other American Indian people in San Francisco and across the United States.

As prayers are offered for the office space to become ceremonial and safe, I can see the members of the group begin to stand closer together. One participant, an older man in his fifties, speaks first. His tone, as he tells of his transition from the reservation in Nevada to urban life in San Francisco, is one of authority. He describes unbelievable trauma and yet there is hope in his message. He recalls a time when San Francisco was a beacon for gay, Two-Spirit, and transgender Natives, but explains that there has since been a decline in leadership within the community. Other participants are nodding in agreement. A transgender participant in her early forties suggests that the only way a community can heal is if it remains a community. I hear the relevance of this insight to HIV prevention efforts: focusing on behavioral change at the individual level causes a greater degree of stigmatization and isolation, which in turn increase harmful behaviors and lead to higher HIV transmission risk.

At the end of the session, I thank each participant and shake their hand, then sit silently in the room, still smelling the remnants of the sage, and ponder the importance of the exchange between the participants. They were asking for a shift from a cultural deprivation model to a healing intervention model, one that examines relationships between people rather than between a disease and an individual. My research has taught me that articulating subjectivities requires humanizing people. Putting the emphasis on humanization in turn underscores the salience of kinship in producing mutual responsibility aᵣ community care, both central principles of decolonization in Indigenous c munities. Interventions founded on kinship act as vehicles for transform' dismantling systems of oppression while reinforcing self-determination. As I listened to the painful stories shared by group participants—stories of sexual violence, rape, racism, sexism, and transphobia, as well as of in-school bullying, family violence, drug abuse, and high-risk sexual behavior—I began to ask more questions about what strategies participants had used in order to cope with these traumas and stressors. It became clear to me over time that love, both self-love and community love, had often been missing from their experiences. It was when they became vulnerable and when they shared stories with one another that they began to see each other as kin, as family—and in seeing one another as kin or family, they became able to find loving connections, based on shared resiliency in the face of colonial trauma.

Over the next year, I would conduct five focus groups and hold dozens of discussions and interviews at the first annual Two-Spirit Powwow at the San Francisco LGBT Center, where hundreds of Native people from across the United States and Canada were in attendance. After more than a year of ethnographic research, I came to the conclusion that to bring meaningful change, an intervention had to come from the participants themselves. Indigenous peoples must be at the center of any decolonial research project—including my own. Making the voices of those most affected central to the discussion is a form of self-determination recognized by scholars and activists across the field of Native studies. What I offer in this empirical work, together with the stories and theoretical analysis shared by the gay men and transgender people in this study, is a handbook of sorts on how the discipline of Indigenous studies can respond to the growing need for empirical research that merges theory and practice, generating reciprocity and solidarity.

This book speaks not only to power and politics in Indigenous studies, but also to the role of the oral tradition in restoring, or at least rejuvenating, a ceremonial practice that I term radical love. The interventions that made this possible may seem small. During each focus group, we offered prayer with sage. We shared meals together before delving into deep dialogue. Participants discussed everything from boarding schools to sexual violence; sharing stories became, for them, a way to build power. Together, these gestures created space for radical love, a methodology for engaging with our own vulnerabilities and mental health struggles. It insists that only when we become vulnerable and open up our hearts to our pain can we truly begin to heal, to sow growth where trauma once stood.

Radical love, as I employ it here, involves a dissolution of boundaries between human beings, wherein a deep sense of love for all aspects of life shatters notions of difference between male, female, queer, Two-Spirit, mixed-race, differently able, et cetera. Patrick Cheng explores the notion of radical love as a deconstruction of social, political, cultural, sexual, and religious boundaries in his book *Radical Love: An Introduction to Queer Theology* (2011). According to Cheng, "God-like queer relationships can be understood as radical love itself. In other words, God is the very manifestation of a love that is so extreme that it dissolves existing boundaries, including the traditional divide between the divine and the human." Radical love challenges the social boundaries that suggest that certain types of love (queer love, Indigenous love, interracial love) are less valid than other types of loving relationships. Moreover, radical love asks us to take personal responsibility for the well-being of those who are most different from us.

When we think of HIV/AIDS today, we must understand that every single person living with the virus has a story. It is my hope that the narratives in *Indian Blood* will speak not just to those in public health and sexuality, but also to those seeking intersectional frameworks for methodological research that repositions language, behavior, and action.

As you read *Indian Blood,* it is my hope that you find it accessible, and much more of a story than an academic project. While I attempt to write for a general audience, the issues surrounding HIV and mixed-race identity within LGBT and Two-Spirit Indigenous communities are not only vast, but highly specific: some issues raised here will be much more familiar to insiders in the field. I welcome those who are less familiar with the fields of American Indian studies, public health, critical mixed-race studies, and queer theory to think deeply, as they read, about the historic and contemporary relationships between Natives and non-Natives. Moreover, I invite all readers to understand that the sometimes highly political nature of my writing is intentional. For far too long, academia has been reluctant to take cultural and political positions that address the very real, everyday needs of the most disadvantaged members of our communities. *Indian Blood* attempts to work against this history, by analyzing contemporary modes of Two-Spirit subjectivity as a reclamation of traditional, non-Western mechanisms for healing, self-love, and decolonization. Finally, I want to acknowledge that this work makes use of a great number of acronyms and new terms. I have included them as part of an effort to bridge differences between public health, mixed-race studies, queer theory, and Indigenous studies. *Indian Blood* attempts to locate an interdisciplinary framework for discussing the multi-identity issues that shape contemporary Native communities. Bridging these seemingly divergent fields requires new ways of thinking, naming, and articulating Native perspectives, requires transforming the language and tools currently available to discuss communities with intersecting and diverse sets of identities. This work seeks to utilize the words, stories, and experiences of Native participants to create a radical discourse. Its aim is Indigenous self-determination in both the formation and dissemination of knowledge systems, in order to transform and improve the lives of American Indians who are mixed-race, queer-identified, transgender, and/or Two-Spirit (MLGBTQ2S) people.

ACKNOWLEDGMENTS

Where do I begin? This book has been in the making for at least six years. Many things have happened along the way to allow this work to become public. It is a work by and for the community, and took many voices, hands, hearts, and minds to create. I will never be able to fully thank the fifty individuals who took part in the research for *Indian Blood*. They each gave of their time, spirit, and heart when they shared often painful and traumatic life stories with me. I am aware of the privilege and responsibility I now carry in holding and sharing their stories. We together created a research ceremony that did not begin and end with the roles of researcher and research participants. We shared meals together and walked together in the community at powwows and other social gatherings. The site of our ceremony was the Native American AIDS Project (NAAP) in San Francisco. The staff demonstrated such love and kindness in their candid discussions with me. They offered extremely helpful feedback and advice throughout the entire process, from recruitment to dissemination back to the community. I will always consider the NAAP staff as members of my own family. My love to Andrew Lopez, Gayle Burns, and Joan Benoit.

I wish to extend my sincere thanks to Ann Auleb, the grandmother of one of my students at Presidio Hill School, where I worked in 2003. Ann was a biology professor at San Francisco State University and through her encouragement I began teaching a course on People of Color and AIDS at SFSU in the spring of 2004. It was in teaching this course that I developed an interest in the intersections between mixed-race identity, sexuality, gender, and HIV. I am very grateful to Ranjit Arab, Brian Folk, Caroline Knapp, Jacqueline Volin, and Jade Brooks for the editorial support and assistance that they offered during the development of the manuscript. Their recommendations, encouragement, and critiques have significantly improved the quality of this book. I remain deeply indebted to them for their belief that this book was an important scholarly and community-based contribution to discussions of decolonization, trauma, and healing through radical love.

I have been fortunate to have many amazing mentors as I developed this project, from grant submissions to conference presentations and to the final research design. My mentors Rafael Diaz, George Ayalya, Jim Wiley, Bonnie

Duran, Karina Walters, Nina Wallerstein, Irene Vernon, Tomas Almaguer, and G. Reginald Daniel have provided me with sound advice and constructive feedback that deeply shapes my thinking about public health, critical mixed-race studies, and the sociology of race and HIV/AIDS. I was also very blessed to receive funding from the Indigenous HIV/AIDS Research Training (IHART) program, a project funded through the National Institutes of Mental Health (Grant R25MH084565) and based at the Indigenous Wellness Research Institute (IWRI) at the University of Washington in Seattle. I am particularly indebted to Karina Walters and Bonnie Duran, the codirectors of the IHART program. Karina and Bonnie's vision has provided so many important opportunities for IHART fellows and Indigenous scholars from across the nation to gain invaluable research and grant-writing skills. They have built a community of scholars, mentors, and scientific leaders at IWRI that is truly groundbreaking in its vision, scope, and innovative design. As their mission statement explains, "IHART aims to develop a network of scholars dedicated to culturally grounded research that will contribute to ameliorating health disparities among American Indians and Alaska Natives (AI/AN)." I encourage other Indigenous and minority scholars to consider this program (http://depts.washington.edu/ihartp/).

IWRI and IHART offered me not only top-notch mentoring from experienced grant writers and researchers, but also an entire team of IWRI and IHART peers and research leaders who assisted me with survey design and data analysis, as well as initial feedback on the theoretical framework for this book. I am forever grateful to the other members of the IHART team who made this research possible: Meg MacDonald, Cynthia Pearson, Jane Simoni, Tessa Evans-Campbell, Michelle Johnson-Jennings, David Patterson, Chris Charles, Jan Beals, Debra Buchwald, David Takeuchi, Julie Baldwin, Geri Doneberg, John Lowe, and Spero Manson. In addition to the IHART family at the University of Washington, my department colleagues in American Indian studies at SFSU—Joanne Barker, Robert Keith Collins, Melissa Nelson, John-Carlos Perea, Gabriela Segovia-McGahan, Amy Lonetree, Clayton Dumont, Jacob Perea, Esther Lucero, Sara Sutler-Cohen, Kathy Wallace, Amy Casselman, Jessica Hope LePak, Eddie Madril, and WeiMing Dariotis (Asian American studies)—have also been a wonderful resource. I am very appreciative of their encouragement of my work for the past fifteen years. In the years leading up to the publication of this manuscript I also received funding and support from the Minority Research Infrastructure Support Program (MRISP) and Research Infrastructure in Minority Institutions (RIMI) grants at SFSU, as well as generous sabbatical funding in the fall of 2013 from provost and vice-president for academic affairs, Sue Rosser. This support, along with that of my college dean and mentor, Kenneth Monteiro, and associate dean Amy Sueyoshi, has allowed me the time away from teaching and administrative duties necessary to finish the research and writing for this book. I also benefitted enormously from the support of three fantastic graduate student research assistants, Haruki Eda, Andrew Millspaugh, and Kei Fischer—your dedication and service to this project and the community is a testament to your belief in the sacred aspects of ceremonial research. I have been very fortunate to have wonderful healthcare in my life and am deeply appreciative of my doctor, Deborah Gold, who has given me the best care, support, and advice that I could have asked for along my journey. Our conversations over the past fourteen years about the HIV epidemic and my research were useful and thought provoking.

To my dear friends in the Native community and beyond, your guidance, support, and enduring love has meant everything in completing this project: Ixayanne Baez, Elton Naswood, Esther Lucero, Rain Gomez, Carolyn Dunn, Tracey Colson-Antee, Jessica Hope LePak, Nazbah Tom, Ann Marie Sayers, Corrina Gould, Carolyn Kualii, Fuifuilupe Niumeitolu, Aidan Dunn, Marcus Arana (Holy Old Man Bull), Jessi Bardill, Miho Kim, Melissa Attia, Oscar Chavez, Rani Marcos, and Vicente Garcia. Much love and gratitude to the Creole Bandits: Melissa Attia, Justin Bernard, Ruben Moreno, and Little Nassima. William Hawk, thank you for our many conversations and moments of laughter as well as the deep thoughts on the most pressing issues facing our communities.

I am above all thankful to my family. They have seen me through so many life challenges over the years. My siblings continue to inspire me with their love of life. They, along with their children, are a constant source of joy. In particular, I want to offer my love and appreciation to my Uncle Charlie, my Aunts Greta, Stephanie, Karen, Sheila, and Carol, my brothers, Eric, Derick, Kevin, Nathan, and Charles, and my sister, Makeba. Time may not heal all wounds, yet the joy from past memories lasts a lifetime. To my cousins Anthony LaChapelle and Trevor Lemond, thank you for being my rock when I needed it most. Johnasies McGraw—thank you for always, always being by my side and for never giving up on me, on us. Our love remains stitched as a sacred remembrance in my mind always. Puleiaava Basil Thomsen, thanks for teaching me that I need to love myself first and for inspiring me to always do better. Alex Trapps-Chabala, you came along at an important time in my life and your kindness, intelligence, and love will always remain close to my heart. To my Australian Aboriginal and Canadian First Nations family, thank you for opening your hearts, traditional lands, and communities to me as I worked on the final stages of this book.

James Ward, Michelle Tobin, Colin Mickelo, Arone Meeks, Jodes Barney, Ed Bennett, James Saunders (and Anthem), Ken Clement, Doris Peltier, Jessica Danforth, Randy Jackson, Marama Pala (Maori, Aoetearoa), Michael Costello, Trevor Stratton, and Lola Forester, I will always feel the connection and love between our ancestors. Dontrey St. Julien, thank you for being my Creole prince in shining armor. In the end, I would be nothing though without my loving and generous first-teachers, my parents, who always demonstrated through their actions how deeply they loved me and how much they wanted me to succeed and contribute something. Even in death, my mother has taught me to keep fighting and working to be the best person that I can be. Since her death in 2012, my father has taught me how to hold onto faith and to those you love. Annetta and Kenneth Jolivette, you are my hope and my inspiration for this work. To the Indigenous women, men, and Two-Spirit people struggling to resist colonial haunting, it is my hope that this work sheds light on your stories as you journey toward decolonization, liberation, and self-determination.

INDIAN BLOOD

CHAPTER 1

Indian Blood

Two-Spirit Return in the Face of Colonial Haunting

My elders told me life was once different before colonists came.
You see in that time we were once accepted and honored.
Then we were vanishing, but now we are coming
back to the ways of our ancestors.

—Indian Blood focus group respondent

AS I RECALL MY INTRODUCTION INTO THE FIELD OF HIV/AIDS AND epidemiology, I remember the important words and research of my mentor Rafael Diaz, author of *Latino Gay Men and HIV* (1997), who wrote, "So many people when they disclose or talk about their HIV status say, 'I'm HIV positive.'" Diaz points out that people with cancer don't say, "I am cancer." They say, "I have cancer." Reframing how we think about HIV/AIDS can shift our well-being as marginalized communities within the capitalist bureaucracy of the public health care system in the United States.

In 2005, in a keynote address for World AIDS Day delivered at San Francisco State University, a mixed-race gay American Indian man stated:

> HIV and AIDS is something that I have learned to live with. It's also something
> that a part of me feels happened for a reason. I wasn't sure if I should disclose
> my status in this way here today. I spoke with a colleague about it and he said,
> "How will disclosing impact you? Will it benefit you? Are you giving anything
> up?" I thought to myself: as a Native gay man of color, I have a responsibility
> to disclose. This is a very personal decision, but in Indigenous communities
> and in communities of color we lack faces to make this pandemic real. If
> you've never known someone living with AIDS, now you do. You know my
> story and in sharing it I hope that others will know that they can live with this.

> They can have a career, a family. They too can find love again. Over the past
> three years I have learned AIDS is not me. I am me. AIDS is only one other
> part of my life.

This man's story is not uncommon. For American Indian people today, HIV/
AIDS, gender, sexuality, and mixed-race identity intersect in complex and traumatic ways in the absence of the community support, cultural buffers, and
stress-coping mechanisms needed to combat colonial oppression.

This is my story, too. I was the one who delivered that keynote talk. As I
reflect back on the eleven years since I first delivered the speech and disclosed
my HIV/AIDS positive status to my colleagues and students, a lot has happened. I think about the scars that living with HIV/AIDS may have left on my
life. I think about the traumas that have existed in my communities for more
than five centuries in the Americas. In 2002, when at the age of twenty-seven
I received my AIDS diagnosis, I had thirty-five T-cells and a viral load of over
five hundred thousand. I truly believed I was at the end of my life, but finding
strength in my own vulnerabilities has allowed me to survive.

A few months after my release from the hospital, twenty-five pounds lighter
and quite fragile, I went to a pipe ceremony and prayer meeting organized by
friends with a medicine man, Daniel Freeland from the Navajo Nation. My
endeavor to write this book, to share these stories, and to seek out a useful
intervention for social and cultural reform stems from the words Dan spoke
to me on that night so many years ago. He said, "You can't think of yourself
as sick. There are a lot of people out there in our communities who are going
through the same thing that you are, and you can tell your story and you can
help them to tell theirs, and in that way you can be a part of the process of
mending the hoop that ties us all together. We don't all get to tell our story,
many have passed on." He continued, "You have to begin to think about what
healing means, what wellness means, and how there is all kinds of medicine
out there. But the greatest medicine is your brother and your sister. You are
your own healing."

Dan's words sum up my own articulation of the concept of radical love, a
primary theme of this book. Socialization and stigmatization in the West create
fractures and forces us to compartmentalize our lives, separating our health,
our education, and our spirituality. Radical love seeks to bring all of these frag-
mented pieces back together. As a critical intervention, it asserts that without
a process of mutual love, respect, and responsibility, we can never truly heal
or achieve self-determination.

Although Cheng (2011) introduced the term radical love in theology and queer studies, it is a new theoretical concept in the context of American Indian studies. An Indigenous framing of radical love, as I define it, stems from a spiritual, cultural, and communal concern for the well-being of all other living things. Radical love in an Indigenous framework embraces all living things as relatives deserving of respect, nurturing, and care, which require in turn an emphasis on physical, spiritual, and emotional health. Radical love by necessity involves a sense of openness and vulnerability, both from community members and from researchers who practice in institutions of higher education.

I open with my own story because I believe in the practice of research justice as an extension of radical love. Research justice is about seeking solidarity with research participants. It is about working with—not on—research participants to weave a narrative, a set of life histories captured in one moment in time. Research justice is a strategic framework and methodological intervention intended to transform structural inequities in research. It insists on the centrality of community voices and leadership, in an effort to facilitate genuine, lasting social change and to foster critical engagement with communities of color, Indigenous peoples, and other marginalized groups. Research justice uses research as an empowering intervention and active disruption of the colonial policies and institutional practices that contribute to the (re)production of social inequalities in research and public policy. It is a ceremonial act that seeks to shift our focus from simple data gathering to relationship building, as a single community formed of scholars, cultural experts, and knowledge keepers. The DataCenter, the organization credited with coining the term, believes that research justice is achieved when marginalized communities are recognized as experts and reclaim, own, and wield *all* forms of knowledge and information (Jolivette 2015). It is within this context, of knowledge construction as a component of research justice, that this book endeavors to engage with multiple forms of Indigenous knowledge and intellectualism.

When I set out to conduct the research for the original pilot study that became *Indian Blood,* I was an IHART (Indigenous HIV/AIDS Research Training) Fellow at the Indigenous Wellness Research Institute at the University of Washington, under the mentorship of Karina Walters and Bonnie Duran. My foray into public health and HIV disparities research—and the methodological framework of this book as a critical intervention into the HIV/AIDS epidemic— is deeply influenced by my experiences both with research justice and with the IHART program. Each offers a vehicle for intervening in the most pressing questions in Native American studies today. First and foremost, the field must ask: How do we understand the contemporary impact of colonial haunting on the well-being of Indigenous peoples?

The concept of colonial haunting, like that of settler colonialism, recognizes the ongoing contemporary impact of colonization on Indigenous peoples (Vernaci 2010, Hixson 2013). Colonial haunting builds on notions of the aftermath and afterlife of violence (Gomez-Barris 2008) and on Avery Gordon's theory of haunting (2008). Many public health scholars discuss the problem of intergenerational trauma in Indigenous communities, but they rarely acknowledge that this trauma stems from a form of spiritual, psychological, cultural, and often metaphysical haunting. I contend that colonial haunting is a contemporary and interconnected web of acts of terror against the minds, bodies, and memories of Indigenous peoples. It produces ruptures in individual and collective methods for coping with stress as well as the social supports, behaviors, and norms that protect individuals and communities from the worst effects of trauma.

Understanding the nature of the colonial haunting that has displaced, removed, relocated, and perpetrated mass acts of genocide (e.g., kidnapping, boarding school abuse, sexual assaults, murder, forced sterilization, etc.) against Indigenous peoples, contributes to our understanding of the significance of what Linda Tuhiwai Smith (1999) has termed "Indigenous methodologies." Smith argues that for most Indigenous peoples in the Americas and the Pacific, because of these historical and ongoing abuses and the lack of access to writing about our own communities, research is considered a "dirty word." Thus, to build a research relationship based on solidarity and research justice, one must consider research as a ceremony.[1] According to Cree scholar Shawn Wilson: "If Indigenous ways of knowing have to be narrowed through one particular lens (which it certainly does not), then surely that lens would be relationality. All things are related and therefore relevant. This concept permeates recent scholarly writings by Indigenous scholars. They question whether, in fact, it is even possible for dominant system researchers to understand this concept with the depth that is required for respectful research with indigenous peoples" (Wilson 2009: 58).

This book contributes to the discourse on research justice as a ceremonial act by examining crucial sites of survival, resistance, and perseverance in the face of trauma, colonial haunting, and HIV disparities within mixed-blood American Indian communities. As a collection of Indigenous voices, this book weaves together the contemporary realities of queer, LGBTQ, and Two-Spirit people, offering new transdisciplinary theories in the hope of interrupting the tragedies of imperialism and colonialism within Indigenous communities in the United States. It is my intention that this work will serve as one of many tools in the arsenal of Indigenous scholars, activists, tribal leaders, and community-based organizations seeking methods for social change, as well as holistic cultural and political change, in the quality of life of Native peoples in North America and beyond. The history of the HIV/AIDS epidemic among Native peoples has been severely understudied (particularly by non-Natives), making this work even more crucial as an intervention tool for the ways we understand the correlations between colonialism, mixed-race identity, and health disparities such as HIV.

Today, HIV/AIDS is no longer considered an automatic death sentence, as it was in the 1980s and early 1990s. But while new advances in HIV/AIDS research continue to reduce mortality rates in the United States, HIV/AIDS continues to disproportionately impact Indigenous communities and little to no research has identified those most at risk for infection, particularly in the most marginalized segments of Native communities. American Indians and Alaska Natives have the third-highest rates of infection after African Americans and Latinos. According to the Centers for Disease Control (CDC 2010) at least 75 percent of HIV infection cases in the Native community involve men who have sex with men.

The CDC identifies several factors specific to American Indian communities that increase the chances for seroconversion (the threshold at which an antibody becomes detectable in the blood, confirming a change in viral infection status from negative to positive). American Indians have the second-highest rate of sexually transmitted infections (STIs) among all ethnic groups; having an STI increases susceptibility to HIV infection. American Indians have higher poverty rates, complete fewer years of education, are younger, are less likely to be employed, and have lower rates of health insurance (CDC 2010)—all factors that limit their access to high-quality health care, housing, and HIV prevention education. High rates of alcohol and drug use, which lead to sexual behaviors associated with increased risk for infection, are other factors leading to increased rates of infection (CDC 2010). Despite the passage of the Affordable Care Act under President Barack Obama, many Native Americans are unlikely to take full advantage of the new provisions, as a result of a long history of mistrust of federal policies. According to a 2013 *USA Today* article, "Although tribal members are entitled to free health care, most Indian health facilities do not offer a full array of services. When patients need major surgery or cancer treatments, for example, they are referred to specialists outside of Indian lands." The article goes on to address how uninsured status increases poor health outcomes and lack of access among American Indian people: "As a group, the nation's

5.2 million Native Americans have poorer health and less access to health care than the rest of the U.S. population. Their uninsured rate is nearly 30 percent, compared to 15 percent for the country as a whole" (Vestal 2013).

Mistrust of the U.S. government and its facilities is a significant barrier to HIV prevention. Indian Health Service (IHS) provides approximately two million American Indians with direct services, including tribally operated and urban Indian health centers. But there continues to be concern about the ability of government-run agencies like IHS to successfully address health dispari-ties in Native communities. Concerns about confidentiality and quality of care, along with a general mistrust toward the U.S. government, cause many Ameri-can Indians to avoid IHS altogether unless they are already quite ill (United States Civil Rights Commission 2004). These low rates of care likely contribute to lower rates of awareness of HIV status in American Indian communities. For example in 2009, 18 percent of those infected with HIV in the general U.S. adult population were unaware of their status, compared with 25 percent among American Indians.

Data limitations in HIV/AIDS research are perhaps the most significant factor responsible for the dearth of scholarship on this subject. American Indi-ans more than any other demographic suffer from extreme underreporting due to racial misclassification (CDC 2012). Racial misidentification of Native people, particularly those of mixed ethnicity (nearly 70 percent of the current population is estimated to be racially mixed) leads to undercounting of this population in HIV surveillance systems and to the underfunding of American Indian-specific prevention programs (U.S. Census 2010).

One of the fastest-growing segments of the U.S. population is people who identify as multiracial. This population has grown by 32 percent since 2000, when the option to check two or more races became available on the U.S. cen-sus. Early data on mixed-race youth and HIV/AIDS suggest that this population may have the highest rates of HIV infection of all groups, though additional research to verify initial trends is necessary (Valleroy, MacKellar, Karon, Rosen, McFarland, Shehan, and Douglas 2000). It is within this context that my research began in 2010, as a collaboration with the Native American AIDS Project in San Francisco, with the goal of better understanding how ethnic-specific health prevention and population-targeted funding can minimize HIV/ AIDS risk among the most at-risk in American Indian communities.

Indian Blood therefore, as a ceremonial act, offers a critical interrogation of the intersections of queer theory, anti-Indianism, critical mixed-race stud-ies, public health, and queer Indigenous community formation. This is the first book to examine the relationship between mixed-race identity and HIV/AIDS.

It is also the first empirical, book-length work to provide an analysis of the emerging and often contested Two-Spirit identity category within the American Indian community as it relates to public health and mixed-race identity. *Indian Blood* is more than an intellectual project—it is a haunting that conjures ghosts from a colonial period spanning more than 520 years in the Americas. It is a collection of the intergenerational memories and traumas relived today among mixed-race, queer-identified, transgender, and Two-Spirit (MLGBTQ2S) American Indians.

Based on surveys, focus groups, and community discussions, this book challenges readers to rethink the connections between identity categories and public health. As subjects-in-process, Two-Spirits, gay and bisexual men, and transgender people in the American Indian community contest rigid colonial and patriarchal narrations regarding blood—both metaphorically, in the case of race and ethnicity, as well as more literally, in the exchange of "blood" during intimate sexual contact.[2] Here "blood" is symbolic of both the politics of racial mixing and the stigmatization of having an "infected" or "diseased" body.

Indian Blood examines colonial and settler colonial repression of Native agency and subjectivity through the development of a psychosocial nexus of HIV risk. The Indian Blood psychosocial nexus of HIV risk model (IBPN HIV risk model) includes six interconnected psychological and social factors that produce high-risk sexual behavior. These six factors are Two-Spirit cultural dissolution, historical and intergenerational trauma, gender and racial discrimination, mixed-race cognitive dissonance, sexual violence, and impaired stress-coping in urban Indian kinship networks.

I argue that as the precontact spiritual, socio-economic, and cultural significance of Two-Spirit individuals have dissolved through colonial contact with Europeans, mixed-blood American Indian queer people have experienced ruptures in the social and cultural support networks that would, under normal circumstances, have served as protective factors. As discrimination against Two-Spirits has increased from contact to the present, it has combined with a breakdown in traditional/tribally specific values, beliefs, and practices that lead to intergenerational trauma. Within the context of the MLGBTQ2S experience, trauma is manifested through racial and gender discrimination, mixed-race cognitive dissonance, and sexual violence. If these traumas are left unaddressed from a diverse range of Two-Spirit cultural ethics, they weaken stress-coping mechanisms within urban Indian kinship networks. The only way to heal from these traumas is through a return to a Two-Spirit cultural ethic of support, intergenerational mentoring, and ceremonial healing.

TWO-SPIRIT BODIES, COLONIAL TRAUMA,
AND HAUNTING IMAGINARIES

Decolonization is a central goal of this book. In order to decolonize gender, sexuality, and mixed-race identity within the American Indian community, we must understand the diversity of terms, practices, beliefs, and traditions that exist today and that were practiced in the past. Literature on the identity development processes of American Indians in terms of gender and sexuality has flourished in recent years (Walters, Evans-Campbell, Simoni, Ronquillo, and Bhuyan 2006; Giley 2006; Driskill 2008; Driskill, Finley, Giley, and Morgensen 2011; Adams and Phillips 2009; and Morgensen 2011). *Indian Blood* seeks to expand upon this emerging body of literature by specifically examining how mixed-race identity impacts gender and sexuality development among Native and Indigenous peoples, especially within urban Indian environments.

In many precolonial tribal societies, American Indian gender identities were much more diverse and complex than those in Western societies (Roscoe 1998). Historically, most anthropological research lacked a full understanding of what today many in academia and within American Indian communities across the United States call "Two-Spirit" people (Jacobs, Thomas, and Lang 1997; Giley 2006). While there are many debates and tensions about who and what counts as "Two-Spirit," there is little doubt that the term emerged in the latter years of the twentieth century in response to colonial repression of Native ontologies of gender and sexuality (Driskill 2008). Qwo-Li Driskill begins that essay on Two-Spiritedness and transformation with this discussion about terms:

> As we assemble, I know that there are non-Cherokees and non-Two-Spirit people who are also with us, listening to this story. I would like to ask our guests to sit and just listen from a distance, understanding that because I'm speaking to other Cherokee Two-Spirits/GLBTQ folks, that there are many questions, issues, and terms that I won't be explaining here. And since I brought up terminology, I would like to say to other Cherokee Two-Spirit people that we need to remember that gender systems before invasion and colonization were not the same as they are now. While we subsume same-sex relationships and gender "nonconformity" under the umbrella of "Two-Spirit," it is difficult to say if these identities were linked together in the past. There are numerous experiences and identities that we shove under terms like "Two-Spirit" or "Queer" or "GLBT." I've heard several different terms to talk about these

identities in Cherokee, but I am going to use "Two-Spirit" as my umbrella term
here, knowing that not all of us use this term for ourselves any more than all
of us use any of the other terms available to us in English. All of these terms
and ideas are slippery and complicated, but "Two-Spirit carries with it a particular commitment to decolonization and Indigenous histories and identities
that is at the center of this particular telling.

As Driskill's remarks suggest, the idea that there are only two genders (male
and female) and only two ways of expressing sexual identity (heterosexual and
homosexual) has never been true for a great many American Indian tribes in
the United States (Jacobs, Thomas, and Lang 1997; Roscoe 1998; Giley 2006).
However, it is important to avoid the temptation to use *Two-Spirit* as a universal
category that represents all Native peoples now or prior to colonial contact, or
to conflate the term with either sexual orientation or gender identity, as Adams
and Phillips (2009) point out that many in academia do. By contrast, both in
historical tribal contexts and in contemporary urban Indian communities, the
definition and usage of the term is much more expansive and has its basis in
cultural practices that dictate diverse sets of gender roles within Indigenous
populations in the United States. The term *Two-Spirit* is becoming an effective tool of empowerment, transformation, and subject-making among many
Indigenous peoples.

One of the major aims of this research is to understand how the term Two-
Spirit is put into contemporary use and practice by American Indians. As we've
seen, the term is contested and I use it here as a *remembering* (Driskill, Finley,
Giley, Morgensen 2011). In this instance, remembering is a way to acknowledge
that how same-sex love, desire, and social behavior were historically experienced impacts our contemporary understanding of Two-Spirit identified people
within Indigenous communities. I am not using Two-Spirit as an umbrella term
or a catchall phrase to represent all the various identities and lived expressions
of gender and sexuality among American Indian people. Two-spirit is not a term
that existed in English prior to contact; it is a relatively recent phenomenon and
yet it exists because some of our people, from some of our tribal communities
and urban pan-Indian communities, remember another way of being—one that
is expansive and open, rather than reductive and closed.

Two-Spirit bodies—those bodies that are deemed to lie outside the normal
gender and sexual identity classifications described and articulated by colonial
powers from 1492 to the present—have been beaten, silenced, and traumatized
in often insurmountable ways. And yet a remembering is taking place among

Native and Indigenous peoples that calls for a reconciliation of all of our parts. This remembering seeks to "heal" our blood in both a metaphoric and a literal sense. Questioning who has "Indian blood" and how one can be "contaminated" by "bad blood" both through disease and through intermarriage to the "wrong type" of racial/ethnic/gendered group is a part of the colonial haunting that continues to pervade Native and Indigenous communities, especially when it comes to issues of authenticity and legitimacy (Sturm 2002, Garroutte 2002, Barker 2012). This ongoing battle over defining Indian blood and, by extension, Indian bodies, is perhaps the greatest trauma, the greatest soul loss/wound that we must address in order to undo the process of Two-Spirit cultural dissolution (Duran and Duran 1995).

Two-spirit bodies experience psychological assault, physical violence, negation, and erasure as a result of colonial and settler-colonial narratives concerning the performance of gender and sexuality within Western categorical definitions. *Indian Blood* asserts that when Two-Spirit people are marked as possessing aberrant, non-normative bodies, their spiritual, mental, and ceremonial protective factors become eroded, and colonial trauma deposits itself as a physical and intergenerational presence, producing a haunting imaginary within contemporary American Indian MLGBTQ2S communities. The effect of this haunting is what Eduardo and Bonnie Duran (1995) describe as soul loss. Haunted subjects experience not only soul loss but also illness and the debilitation of community networks of support, which in turn cause a dissolution of a Two-Spirit ethic of mutual respect and reciprocity.

Duran and Duran's discussion of illness and its connection to soul loss provides a starting point for my assertion that spirit trauma is a specific form of psychological and emotional injury that causes a loss of one's culturally specific stress-coping mechanisms—all within the context of settler colonial displacement, ethnic erasure, and loss of viable kinship support networks. "One cause of the illness," they write "is the departure of the soul from the body. The second possible cause of this illness is the theft or abduction of the soul by ghosts or sorcerers. The treatment for this illness comes through the restoration of the soul by the healer. Of the traditional concepts, soul loss may be the most difficult for the Western worldview to accept" (Duran and Duran 1995: 20). Soul loss through colonial haunting is an ongoing project of colonization. Linking soul loss to colonial haunting reveals connections between settler colonialism, with its social and economic displacement, and contemporary forms of spiritual conquest and intergenerational trauma as discussed in particular by Native feminist and sovereignty scholars (Alfred 2009; Barker 2005, 2011; Goeman

2013; Simpson 2013; Simpson 2014). This soul loss is similar to spirit-trauma, in that both cause mental and spiritual ruptures in self-esteem and culturally specific understandings of healing, wellness, and stress-coping mechanisms. Soul loss occurs when, as Leanne Simpson's (2013) work suggests, Natives struggle within the spaces of urban and reservation life, where cultural assimilation leads to a diminishing of self-awareness, agency, and Indigenous, First Nation ethnic specificity. Soul loss occurs every day on reservations and in urban spaces in which Native gender, ethnic, and sexual expressions of diversity that counter Western narrations are rendered mute, both by non-Native and Native institutional systems. Circe Sturm's 2002 account of racial identity among the Cherokee Nation suggests that the competing definitions of race as nation and race as blood quantum emerged as a means of defining Cherokee racial and ethnic identity through blood and kinship. This occurred in ways that were deeply impacted by contact with Western colonial powers, whose influence shifted Cherokee thinking about ethnic/racial/national identity.

> In this context of nation building, two competing definitions of race came to shape Cherokee politics and identity in profound ways. The first ideology—race as nation—suggested that race, or racial metaphors of blood and kinship, could be used to define nation "as collective" subject, as a superorganism with a unique biological-cultural essence. The second ideology—race as blood quantum—was buttressed by nineteenth-century scientific thought. It held that blood quantum was a rational measure of racial identity and that the social and biological "fitness" of Native American mixed-bloods could be calculated according to their degree and type of racial mixture. (Sturm 2002: 53)

I argue that representations of MLGBTQ2S identities across Indian Country attempt to suggest that there were no gay Indians prior to colonial contact (see Giley 2006). To accept Two-Spirit, LGBTQ, mixed-race Natives is to accept multiple forms of marginalization, thereby threatening a particular form of tribal nationalism and urban Indian nationalism, one that imagines a tradition which did not always include a diverse group of tribal citizens who were always already mixed-blood, Two-Spirit, and/or LGBT. While the term *Two-Spirit* emerges out of the efforts of LGBT American Indians in the late 1980s to mid-1990s to contest the very limited typologies of sexual identity (e.g., the Cass Model; see Cass 1979), debate and tension continue about the usage of the term to represent a broad and diverse set of identities within the American Indian community, particularly its relationships with tribal nation distinctiveness and linguistic inconsistency, as well as problems centering on gender and sexual identity conflation.[3] To understand the demographics of the research participants in this study, it is important to note that most of the models that attempt to explain sexual identity patterns do not include nor reflect the tribally specific contexts out of which many of the participants emerge. Identification as Two-Spirit or LGBTQ has as much to do with cultural upbringing and Indigenous worldviews as it does with social norms around sexual orientation development models described by Western, non-Native scholars. In order to better understand the impact of cultural upbringing and Indigenous worldviews on the participants, a demographic profile survey was distributed. Its results offer a better understanding of the life stories and cultural influences that impact mixed-race, LGBTQ, and Two-Spirit-identified Natives in the San Francisco Bay Area.

DEMOGRAPHIC PROFILE OF INDIAN BLOOD PARTICIPANTS

It is ironic that the term *Two-Spirit* came into usage to address the fixed and rigid structure of sexuality and gender categories constructed by the West, because today some people within the community believe that the term is either being co-opted by non-Natives or being used to identify all people who are gay, lesbian, bisexual or transgender identified. But as with any identity category, it all depends upon how we seek to use and understand the term Two-Spirit, while not forcing the label on every member of a group with any shared attributes or behaviors. In the summer of 2010 I contacted Native American AIDS Project (NAAP) executive director Joan Benoit about conducting a study on the impact of mixed-race identity on HIV prevalence rates among the American Indian population in San Francisco. Joan agreed to allow me to recruit participants from the NAAP community, but because she was on a sabbatical she put me in contact with Gayle Burns, a respected elder who ran the transgender and women's talking circles at NAAP, to set up the recruitment plan. Gayle and I spoke for a few hours about the goals of the study and why I was involved in HIV work in the American Indian community. We found we had in common our concern about the lack of studies dealing with Natives and HIV and more specifically on mixed-blood Natives and HIV. Through these conversations, my initial plan to only focus on mixed-race gay men shifted to include self-identified transgender people as well. Gayle and Andru Lopez (who led the men's talking circle) helped me to understand the agency's concern about growing rates of violence, sexual abuse, and HIV transmission among transgender Natives. The three of us agreed to host all focus groups on site at NAAP in the evening, to allow participants an opportunity to attend after work. Gayle and Andru agreed to help with recruitment efforts by passing out flyers at local powwows and health and wellness fairs where they would be sharing general information about NAAP and providing free, rapid HIV/AIDS testing. Over the next year, I conducted the five focus groups at NAAP that provide the empirical data for this book.

The participants in this study self-identified their genders and sexual orientations. Among the fifty participants, 66 percent described their gender as male, 14 percent as transgender, 14 percent as Two-Spirit, 4 percent as female, and 2 percent as intersex. Gender self-identification options were intentionally left vague in order to allow transgender people a choice between identifying as male, female, or transgender. The self-identification of the participants demonstrates the diverse range in gender identities among the group and, while reflective of the urban Indian community in the San Francisco Bay Area, it is also suggestive of an ever-diversifying population that refuses to submit to Western colonial standards of gender and sexual identity categories. Breaking down self-identification further in terms of sexual orientation, 64 percent identified as gay/queer, 18 percent as bisexual, and 18 percent as Two-Spirit.

In terms of employment, 16 percent of the participants were students and 34 percent were homeless, retired, unemployed, disabled and/or lived on SSI at the time of the study. The largest share, 44 percent, worked in professional or semi-professional capacities, including education, counseling, health, retail, food services, transportation, insurance, cosmetology, and entertainment. Another 6 percent of respondents did not answer the question pertaining to employment status. The majority, 54 percent, of participants resided in San Francisco, and in other Bay Area cities: 6 percent in Oakland, 4 percent in Antioch, and 4 percent in Oakley. Other cities in the Bay Area (Berkeley, Richmond, San Jose, Vallejo, and Walnut Creek) and beyond (Beaverton, Oregon; El Paso; Indian Canyon, California; Minneapolis; Muskogee, Oklahoma; Phoenix; Portland; Seattle; Tempe, Arizona; and Tulsa) each accounted for 2 percent of respondents. Another 2 percent of participants did not respond to the question about their city of residence. In addition to basic survey questions about employment, race, gender, and residency, participants were also asked their HIV status: 28 percent of respondents stated that they were HIV positive at the time of the study, while the remaining 72 percent reported being negative for the HIV virus. This data was entirely based upon self-reporting; no testing measures were used to verify the HIV status of the participants.

When asked about their tribal affiliation (participants were allowed to report more than one tribal affiliation), 10 percent of participants identified as Apache, 10 percent as Dine/Navajo, 10 percent as Cherokee, 6 percent as Lakota, 4 percent as Anishinaabe/Ojibwa/Chippewa, 4 percent as Arapahoe, 4 percent as Osage, and 4 percent as Pomo. The following tribes were also represented, with 2 percent of participants identifying with each of the respective categories: Blackfeet/Ohlone, Blackfeet, Chickasaw, Choctaw, Cree, Creek, Dakota, Hoopa, Huichol, Kawerak, Mandan, Mestizo, Micmac and Wabanaki, Naya Ji, Ohlone, Paiute, Pima, Sac and Fox/Anishinaabe, and Tepetuan. The final 10 percent stated that their tribal background was either unknown or that they were unsure.

The histories and experiences of this group of participants are vastly diverse, as their tribal affiliations and work backgrounds make clear. This study is not an attempt to over generalize the experiences of all mixed-race American Indians, nor those of all Native people who identify as LGBTQ or Two-Spirit. It is, however, a study about the often discordant and contested genealogies of American Indian gender and sexuality. The population that made up the study represented the largest tribal nations in the country and included members of both recognized and unrecognized tribes. The class, education, and ethnic makeup of the group was extremely diverse, making for a rich data set that reveals much about mixed-blood urban Indian communities.

DISCORDANT AND CONTESTED GENEALOGIES OF AMERICAN INDIAN GENDER AND SEXUALITY

The diversity of the participant sample reflects broader differences between members of the American Indian community. As Scott Morgensen (2011) argues in *Spaces between Us*, to thoroughly understand the impact and material force of settler colonialism on queer and Two-Spirit Native subjects, we must link theories of "Native," "settler," and "queer," envisaging the mutually co-constitutive processes of queer Native identity formation as they function in a contemporary national and global context. In other words, how we understand MLGBTQ2S American Indian history is dependent upon our understanding of how settler colonialism produces the modern queer subject, both Native and non-Native, in the United States. The discordant and contested genealogies of queer, Two-Spirit, mixed-race American Indians can only be comprehended if analyzed within the context of colonial and neocolonial political projects that seek to define queerness.

Native and non-Native people are continually working to make meaning out of simultaneous queer and Indigenous identities, in ways that can weaken or obfuscate the subjectivity of the MLGBTQ2S Native community by basing Native identities on relationships with Europeans and other non-Natives. The question that Morgensen's work raises for me is how we can understand the coexisting histories and narrations of queer Native and queer non-Native people without sacrificing the subjectivities of the queer Native mixed-race subject. These questions only surface as a result of Morgensen's astute analysis that interaction between settler colonialists and Native people produce a particular set of queer Native narratives, ones reinscribed by both Native and non-Native people. I contend, based in part on settler colonial scholarship, that a complex, ongoing colonial haunting negatively affects theories of self within queer, Two-Spirit, and mixed-race, LGBT Native contexts (Alfred 2009; Barker 2005, 2011; Goeman 2013; Simpson 2013; Simpson 2014).

Contact with Europeans, with white Americans, and particularly with white American anthropologists has directly shaped the discordant and contested definitions of American Indian sexuality and gender for more than five hundred years. Early anthropological studies misunderstood the complex and diverse variations in gender and sexuality among Native American tribes and communities throughout the Americas (Jacobs, Thomas, and Lang 1997; Roscoe 2000). The plethora of early anthropological studies on Indigenous sexuality and gender identities have reduced rather than expanded scholarly understanding of Native American culture, behavior, and social interaction within Native and non-Native communities. While these studies reduce the complexity of sexuality and gender among male Two-Spirits, they in large part ignore the roles and experiences of female Two-Spirits. In the case of both male and female Two-Spirits, "homosexuality" and the construction of the "berdache" identity are favored as ways of producing "deviant" "subcultures" within American Indian tribes and communities (Jacobs, Lang, and Thomas 1997: 100).

This anthropological power—to name and narrate alternative ways of practicing and living gendered lives in contradistinction to European mores and values—has had the effect of reproducing inequality within contemporary Native American societies, where MLGBTQ2S people are often ostracized within their own communities. Despite the acceptance and internalization of Western beliefs and values about the diversity of gender and sexual identities within some tribal and urban Indian communities, substantial scholarly evidence suggests that not only has there always been tremendous gender and sexual diversity in Indigenous communities in the United States but also that these identities are based upon much more than sexual behavior (Jacobs, Lang, and Thomas 1997; Roscoe 2000). Furthermore, these roles and gender/sexual expressions were historically integrated, accepted, and valued in most cases.[4] Jacobs, Thomas, and Lang assert that "in many Native American cultures there existed—and in a number of cases still exists—three or four genders: women, men, Two-Spirit womanly males, and less frequently, Two-Spirit/manly females. In each Native American culture that acknowledges multiple genders there also exists specific words to refer to people who are of a gender other than woman or man. Terms referring to Two-Spirit people in Native American languages usually indicate that they are seen as combining the masculine and feminine" (103–4).

Today, effectively disentangling the discordant and contested meanings of Native sexuality and gender within the context of settler colonialism, biopower, and heteropatriarchy is challenging (Finley 2011). The field of Native studies often ignores sexuality, while queer/sexuality studies often ignores racism and cultural difference within scholarship related to Indigenous peoples. At stake in mapping alternative and diverse genealogies of American Indian gender and sexuality are questions of tribal sovereignty and community cohesion. How can a people so traumatically impacted by colonial haunting, genocide, and identity theft remain if their own epistemological ways of being are continually policed, not just by non-Natives but also by their own people? The commentaries that study participants made about the politics surrounding "Indian blood" articulate a way of existing in the world with multiple identities. These identities cannot be separated: race/ethnicity, gender, and sexuality are important aspects not just of identity, but also of self-determination. In order to move toward an active process of decolonization, Indigenous peoples must move away from binaries. These binaries are deeply entrenched in blood quantum, heteronormative citizenship, as well as in an oppressive internal colonial system that weakens tribal sovereignty and inclusivity (Sturm 2002, Garroutte 2002). To break the cycle of colonial haunting and its power in producing discordant and contested understandings of contemporary queer, mixed-race, and Two-Spirit lived experiences, we must also deconstruct heteropatriarchy and heteronormativity within urban Indian and tribal nation-state contexts, since both serve as vehicles for reproducing colonial power within both Native and non-Native communities. Finley (2011) argues that "the simple inclusion of queer people or of sexuality as topics of discussion in Native studies and in Native communities is not enough to effectively detangle the web of colonialism and heteropatriarchy. Taking sexuality seriously as a logic of colonial power has the potential to further decolonize Native studies and Native communities by exposing the hidden ways that Native communities have been colonized and have internalized colonialism" (32).

The correlations between mixed-race identity and blood quantum on the one hand with heteropatriarchy and heteronormativity on the other inform many of the ways that MLGBTQ2S Native individuals are treated within their families and communities. Many turn to high-risk behaviors to mitigate the stress, trauma, and a lack of belonging caused by these psychosocial factors. *Indian Blood* attempts to reweave the broken relationships between Indian communities, both tribal and urban, and MLGBTQ2S people who are at high risk for HIV infection. The pathway to reweaving these relationships involves a mutual process of intergenerational healing, mentorship, and active leadership to thwart and dispel ongoing definitions of Native peoples through colonial eyes. Intergenerational mentoring and cultural leadership among MLGBTQ2S American Indians seeks to restore epistemological understandings of gender, ethnic, cultural, and sexual diversity within tribal and urban Indian communities where "authentic" Native American identities and practices are discordant and contested.

AMERICAN INDIAN SOCIAL MOVEMENTS
AND THE QUESTION OF AUTHENTICITY

Enrollment is a source of ongoing and longstanding debates and tensions within the field of American Indian/Indigenous studies. Issues of "authenticity," whether based on ethnic/racial, gender, or sexual orientation identity categories, often serve only to create conflict and intra-group turmoil rather than to strengthen group cohesion. There is a long history of factionalism within American Indian movements at the local, national, tribal, subtribal, and supratribal levels (Cornell 1990). Concerns about "fake," "impostor," or "wanabee" Indians have been prevalent throughout Indian Country during the twentieth and twenty-first centuries (Cornell 1990, Nagel 1997, Garroutte 2002). Questions about who belongs and who does not are never limited to race and ethnicity. There is also serious tension within the queer, LGBT, Two-Spirit community regarding usage of the Two-Spirit label by potential outsiders appropriating Native cultural worldviews without a thorough or specific tribal ancestral understanding of the complexity of Native gender and sexuality-based identities in their political and ceremonial contexts. Many Native and Indigenous peoples are guarded against individuals who encroach upon Native identities and subjectivities—and with good reason. There is a long history of cultural appropriation and misuse of tribal status in religion, art, law, film, and society at-large. Meanwhile, many American Indians, both on the reservation and within urban areas, continue to live in very difficult conditions, with limited access to economic mobility.

In the context of these tensions and controversies, the selection criteria for participation in the Indian Blood study required that all participants

> Be between the ages of twenty and sixty-five,
>
> Be sexually active, and
>
> Have biological parents or grandparents from multiple racial/ethnic backgrounds, or self-identify as mixed-race and Native American.

They also needed to be either

> Men who have sex with men (MSM) or who self-identify as gay, or
>
> Individuals who identify as transgender, bisexual, and/or Two-Spirit

Many participants have been involved in a range of social movements and community organizing activities. Their involvement in organizations such as Bay Area American Indian Two-Spirits (BAAITS) and Gay American Indians (GAI) makes this group important for understanding the complex and politically contested terrain of contemporary American Indian organizing and social justice activism in the San Francisco Bay Area. Despite the challenges of fulfilling "authenticity" criteria such as minimum blood quantum, tribal enrollment, and possession of a Certificate of Degree of Indian Blood (CDIB), many of the participants still engaged with the American Indian community. This project is first and foremost about collective action and participation, rather than about meeting the racial, sexual, and gendered ascription models produced by Western colonial haunting as well as by the laws and policies created by the U.S. government to limit and destroy the existence of Native and Indigenous peoples.

The book argues that as Native MLGBTQ2S people engage in struggles to (re)claim their place within urban Indian and tribal communities, many refuse to be denied their identities and their right to participate in social justice movements simply on the basis of "authenticity" tests. But even within the study's participants, there was ambivalence about such testing. As one Cherokee participant with experience with both American Indian and Two-Spirit organizations explained that, although "it isn't always popular to bring up,"

When it comes to the leadership roles within an organization, like the board or whatever, I think there should be somehow a majority of people, if it's an Indian organization, that—they should be enrolled. Not that other people who are not enrolled should not be on the board . . . I just think they should be included, but I think the majority of people should always be enrolled. . . . Because I often feel that sometimes you go to an Indian organization with a lot of mixed people and these people who really have very tenuous connections to their Indian identity, because they are mixed. They don't really know the culture of their tribes. If there's gonna be a mixture of people who are enrolled and unenrolled, there's always going to be a majority of the group who are unenrolled. And if they are gonna dominate that group, it's not going to be a space where tribally enrolled people with connections to their cultural identities are going to feel welcomed. They are gonna think, oh this is a bunch of white people who are trying to be Indian, or they're just like . . . fake Indians.

The concerns raised here are strongly felt but miss the point that in California a great many tribes do not have federal recognition, with the result that thousands of tribal members may never be enrolled. *Indian Blood* allows us to understand that the politics of "blood" and "authenticity" only serve to further colonial haunting while simultaneously weakening calls for greater tribal sovereignty and self-determination.

Throughout the 1970s and 1980s, gay American Indians and those who were starting to define themselves as Two-Spirit set the groundwork for contemporary organizing in MLGBTQ2S communities across North America. The challenge today is that there is a generational gap in leadership within the MLGBTQ2S American Indian population. The participants in this book spoke about their concerns for the future because few younger people are taking up leadership positions, in an era of intensifying neocolonial policies that attack the rights and self-determination of MLGBTQ2S American Indians. According to Scott Morgensen (2011), urban relocation and migration in the 1970s was responsible for creating gay American Indian leadership nationally:

GAI members set up booths at powwows and other Native community events (at times in the face of harassment); published testimonies in Native media; and directed Native health programs to address their experiences with AIDS. GAI also sought to educate civic agencies and the broader gay and lesbian movement about their existence and their claim of a historical place in Native nations. According to Randy Burns and Erna Pahe, GAI's visibility persuaded

skeptical urban Indian organizations to later seek GAI out owing to its ties to
the media, government, and social movements. (Morgensen 2011: 78)

In the wake of the successes of organizations like GAI there have also been
new responses from the academic world concerning the existence of queer,
Native Americans. *Living the Spirit* (Roscoe 1988) was a seminal work, the
first to thoroughly give voice to queer/LGBT, Two-Spirit, and some mixed-race
American Indian voices within academia and community organizing. It uses
poetry, testimonials, and history to tell a different story about queer Native
people and it is often cited as the first text to be written largely by gay American
Indians. Since the publication of this anthology, there has been an expansion of
MLGBTQ2S organizing within Native and Indigenous communities. In the San
Francisco Bay Area, the site of this study, there has been a significant increase
in the visibility of MLGBTQ2S American Indians in Pride parades, public hear-
ings (such as the Human Rights Commission's Forum on the status of Native
American people in San Francisco in 2007), conferences, and powwows.

Despite the increasing visibility of this diverse and complex population,
there has also been a decline in local, state, and federal funding to support
the work of cultural competency in health care and other social services. One
painful example of this decline can be found in the competition that is often
created between American Indian health service organizations and nonprofits.
This competition causes agencies to fight for the small pool of resources that
are available locally to Native American community-based organizations. This
competition for resources was responsible in many ways for the recent closing
of the NAAP in December 2012, which did not receive its usual funding from the
City of San Francisco. NAAP's board released the following statement regarding the closure:

> Since 1994, NAAP has provided culturally appropriate direct services to peo-
> ple living with HIV/AIDS as well as HIV prevention programs to people who
> identify as American Indian/Alaskan Native. The staff at NAAP has developed
> many unique and culturally relevant education and support services, which
> have been replicated by other AIDS service organizations. NAAP's staff and
> board would like to thank the individuals and organizations that have sup-
> ported us over the past eighteen years. We could never have completed this
> amazing journey without our entire community. NAAP's staff has worked tire-
> lessly to provide outstanding services to their clients, at times, when budget
> crises arose, even forgoing financial compensation for their work. Because of

this love and support, clients consider NAAP's staff to be family and NAAP's office a home away from home.

As noted earlier, NAAP was my primary organizational partner in this study. They assisted me in the recruitment of participants and served as the host site for all five of the focus group discussions. With the Native American Health Center and the Asian Pacific Islander Wellness Center, it was one of only three ethnic-specific and culturally competent HIV/AIDS service organizations able to meet the needs of the aging, and growing, MLGBTQ2S American Indian population in the San Francisco Bay Area.

NAAP's decline is a direct result of the failure of public policy and government-based funding programs to recognize the correlations between high-risk behavior, ethnic identity, and sociocultural factors. *Indian Blood* argues that Indigenous people's work toward decolonization as a global project must entail strengthening academic and community relationships between the fields of public health, sexuality studies, and Native American studies, if we are to produce a social movement that will allow us to keep proportional rates of HIV/AIDS infection low within this population.

QUEERING PUBLIC HEALTH AND ETHNIC STUDIES DISCOURSE

The loss of organizations like NAAP is significant in the fight against HIV/AIDS. The complexity of MLGBTQ2S American Indian identity makes it extremely difficult for scholars of ethnic studies and public health to fully address the relationships that exist between their intersecting identities. In fact most national health studies fail to record the statistical impact of certain diseases on mixed-race people and American Indians because in the United States, researchers continue to base their research on a binary racial system (between Blacks and whites), although that system is slowly turning into a ternary racial system (white, Black, and Hispanic).

The HIV/AIDS epidemic continues to ravage communities of color at an alarming rate more than thirty years after the onset of the disease. What is most alarming about the current data is that mixed-race gay men aged fifteen to twenty-two have one of the highest HIV incidence rates (Valleroy, MacKellar, Karon, Rosen, McFarland, Shehan, and Douglas 2000). The Valleroy study was conducted because, though HIV studies carried out in the late 1980s suggested that the epidemic had peaked, studies focused on young MSM throughout the

1990s suggested that they continued to have a high HIV incidence rate. The seven-city study not only revealed alarmingly high rates of infection among African Americans as well as among Hispanics, but also was the first national study to demonstrate that men of mixed racial backgrounds (two or more races) were at higher risk for HIV than others. These findings underscore the need to conduct more empirical research on the factors impacting high HIV rates among African American, Hispanic, and mixed-race men. While there has been an increase in the number of studies examining HIV infection rates among African American and Hispanic men, there is still a dearth of empirical data on the current status of the epidemic among mixed-race men. This suggests that new cases of HIV infection can be expected within this population if no primary research is done to understand what is putting this population at risk and what it might take to stop this disease from continuing to be a "silent" killer of multiracial people. It also suggests that more research needs to be done on mixed-race transgender people and their lived experiences as they relate to HIV/AIDS.

Centers for Disease Control (CDC) reports from 2010 underscore the salience of health disparities for youth of color, but lack an analysis of the risks faced by mixed-heritage people. We know that youth of color are particularly vulnerable in all areas of health disparities. In the case of HIV/AIDS, ethnic minority youth are the hardest hit by the HIV/AIDS epidemic, comprising 84 percent of new HIV infections in young people between the ages of thirteen and nineteen (CDC 2010). Youth of color also have disproportionate rates of sexually transmitted infections (STIs), according to the CDC.

The current public health and ethnic studies research literature fails, however, to examine how mixed-race populations experience the impacts of poverty, invisibility, and marginalization within the healthcare system. The leading articles that reference racial and ethnic disparities in the healthcare system do not reveal how the mixed-race population compares to other minority populations in terms of health risk. There is no explanation as to why multiracial youth are more likely to engage in substance abuse or violence or what types of mental health services they may need to reduce these risk behaviors (Choi, Harachi, Gillmore, and Catalano 2006). We only know from this research that mixed-race youth do face racial and ethnic discrimination in schools and in obtaining culturally competent mental health treatment services. There is no qualitative research data on the health and sexual practices of mixed-race gay men, nor among mixed-race people who also identify as transgender, Two-Spirit, or bisexual.

Urgent and life-threatening health disparities are on the rise, particularly in communities of color and among Indigenous peoples. It is difficult to take up a study on mixed-race people and HIV, not only because there is so little data on this subject but also because there are many different racial/ethnic mixtures. Because of this complexity, I chose to focus on mixed-race American Indians because they have the highest rates of interracial marriage (Lee and Edmonston 2005) and they are one of the least-studied populations in the United States. Another challenge in writing this book is the limited existing data and analysis about the needs of mixed-race LGBT individuals within the healthcare system and whether or not mixed-race people experience the same disparities as people of color who identify as monoracial. One could argue that health disparities in communities of color and among Indigenous people are a new form of cultural and ethnic genocide that have unique impact on MLGBTQ2S populations.

While there has been a growing body of research and qualitative data on the lived experiences of people of color, including MSM dating patterns, we only have *one* research datum on mixed-race gay men, focused on HIV prevalence (Valleroy, MacKellar, Karon, Rosen, McFarland, Shehan, and Douglas 2000). However, there is no indication of how many of these men identified as gay men because Valleroy uses the MSM category, nor is there any qualitative data about what is putting these men at risk. Current research does not include any discussion of the sexual behaviors that could be putting mixed-race, queer-identified people at risk for HIV infection.

Indian Blood builds upon the theories of Rafael Diaz (1997) and Cathy Cohen (1999) in arguing that, in considering behavior patterns that are rooted in social factors like homophobia, racial discrimination, poverty, and class, we must first address sociocultural and psychological risk (Diaz 1997). I also consider how Cathy Cohen's articulation of secondary marginalization can explain the lack of research on the experiences of MLGBTQ2S American Indians in the San Francisco Bay Area. Cohen argues that historically speaking, political issues in the Black community have been addressed through what she calls consensus issues. Consensus issues are framed as somehow important to every member of the Black community, either directly or symbolically. These issues, according to Cohen, are often the most visible segments of any Black political agenda, and they often receive the bulk of resources and attention from Black political leaders and organizations. In actuality, she argues, both inside and outside Black communities, certain segments of the population are privileged with regard to the definition of political agendas. For example, issues affecting men are often represented as representative of the condition of an entire community and thus worthy of a group response.

In contrast to consensus issues, cross-cutting political issues involve those concerns which disproportionately and directly affect only certain segments of a marginal group. These issues stand in contrast to consensus issues, she argues, which are understood to constrain or oppress with equal probability all known marginal group members. Cohen argues that the experiences of intravenous drug users, gays and lesbians, and those living with HIV and AIDS are seen as secondary or cross-cutting issues. She asserts that when we only focus on consensus issues, we leave out the most vulnerable members of our communities, causing secondary marginalization: exclusion or invisibility by both mainstream U.S. society and by nonwhite ethnic and racial group(s). For American Indian MLGBTQ2S people, what I term "triple marginalization"—of color, of mixed-race identity, and of LGBTQ2S status—has real consequences for increasing the spread of HIV/AIDS as well as for increasing the associated risk behaviors for contracting the virus.

Given the arguments of both Diaz and Cohen, the work of Valleroy and her colleagues becomes all the more important as a rationale for studying the lived experiences of MLGBTQ2S American Indians. Valleroy's study informs us that mixed-race young men have the second-highest prevalence and highest incidence rates of HIV when compared to other MSM of color. In order to fully understand this sociological phenomenon, an extensive mixed-method study needed to be conducted to focus on the possible correlation between mixed-race identity and HIV/AIDS risk behavior. The literature to date has focused heavily on quantitative studies without gathering qualitative information from self-identified, MLGBTQ2S people. *Indian Blood* takes up the question of whether mixed-race, queer populations experience what I term triple marginalization, as people of color, queer, and mixed-race.

With this challenge as a starting point, the stories included in this book attempt to address a long history of colonial haunting and trauma, as well as the interrelated psychosocial factors that produce high-risk behavior and potentially weak or eroded stress-coping mechanisms and protective factors against HIV transmission. The goal of this book is to identify key factors and variables that impact high-risk sexual behavior in the experiences of MLGBTQ2S American Indians in the San Francisco Bay Area. The book also seeks to offer new policy recommendations and interventions that include more direct services for MLGBTQ2S American Indians in urban environments such as the San Francisco Bay Area. While these stories only speak to a limited and small segment of this specific population, they do provide a basis to inform future studies examining the correlation between mixed-race identity, sexuality, and health disparities.

The pain and trauma the participants have experienced across the course of their lifetimes is revealing. Like the young mixed-race students in Choi's study, these individuals also demonstrate the signs of having gone through many years of abuse, both mental and physical. Therefore, it is imperative that we find new models to disrupt the experience of colonial haunting and Two-Spirit dissolution that has allowed many MLGBTQ2S American Indians to "normalize" or internalize their abuse as either their "fault" or a "natural" product of the society in which we live. Consider the following statement by one of the participants:

> Well, I was initiated into the club at seven, by one of my cousins. And then one of my brother's friends when I was in high school—one of the macho gang guys, like, had his way with me. I was like a good Mormon boy. I wasn't gonna do anything. I already knew I was gay. Everybody knew I was gay. But I was a good little Mormon then. I didn't do anything, I didn't. . . . People at church never said anything. People at school never said anything. But people where we lived, they knew. 'Cause my brother was like, "He's gay. He's a sissy." 'Cause no one would know, outwardly. . . . In my white shirt, and my tie, and my little slacks and my book of Mormon. Nope, I never did anything bad. I was babysitting his sister, [the macho gang guy's] little sister, and I was coming back from school through the field. And he caught me behind the barn. . . . He did things that I actually did like. . . . But I didn't want to do because I was a gay Mormon boy."

Here we can see the participant's "acceptance" of his sexual orientation at a young age, but we also can observe some degree of "acceptance" of the abuse he endured as something "natural," something the respondent could not—and others would not—"do anything" to prevent. Through the course of the research such stories were common, and it became painfully clear that they had to be told. The intersections between gender, race, and sexuality as individual and collective colonial constructs must be decolonized, and what follows is an attempt to open up a dialogue toward that end.

ABOUT THIS BOOK

The Indian Blood psychosocial nexus of HIV risk model (IBPN HIV risk model) includes six interconnected psychological and social factors that produce high-risk sexual behavior: Two-Spirit cultural dissolution, historical and intergenerational trauma, gender and racial discrimination, mixed-race cognitive dissonance, sexual violence, and stress-coping in urban Indian kinship networks. Each chapter takes up a different aspect of the IBPN HIV risk model, piecing together a new research framework for articulating the diversity of American Indian gender, sexuality, and ethnic identities in urban Indian environments. Each chapter also identifies and documents the ways that each psychosocial factor relates to the others to produce an interlocking system of trauma and oppression.

This research began as an attempt to understand the differences between ethnic-specific HIV/AIDS service organizations in comparison to nonethnic-specific agencies, but I quickly learned that there was an important set of stories that lay underneath the HIV service narrative. The participants in this story spoke about their pain, the root cause of much of that pain, and how they believed it could be different if the communities they came from were also different. In responding to these stories, *Indian Blood* becomes a much more powerful story of ceremonial return. Ceremony can happen in many ways and in very simple daily acts. The participants reveal through their own stress-coping strategies and through urban Indian kinship networks that they engage in ceremony almost every day of their lives. *Indian Blood* asserts that we must pursue research agendas that examine the unique challenges facing queer people of mixed ethnicity in the U.S. public health sector.

Chapter 2, "Two-Spirit Cultural Dissolution: HIV and Healing among Mixed-Race American Indians," outlines and describes the IBPN HIV risk model by addressing the origins of Two-Spirit people and how their roles have changed over time in both tribal and urban Indian contexts as a result of colonial contact and ongoing discrimination. The chapter also briefly introduces the intergenerational healing and cultural leadership intervention model (IHCL), a method of addressing the six interrelated psychosocial risk factors for HIV among MLG-BTQ2S American Indians.

Chapter 3, "Historical/Intergenerational Trauma and Radical Love," asserts that as Two-Spirit cultural dissolution takes place, the historical traumas faced by Two-Spirit people—and by extension among all Native people—produce an intergenerational soul wound that cause severe acts of family trauma, abuse, neglect, and internalized oppression to proliferate. Despite centuries of what I term posttraumatic invasion syndrome (PTIS), MLGBTQ2S American Indians are fighting to end triple marginalization through acts of radical love. Radical love is defined by community participation and cultural revitalization activities that take shape through mentoring, leadership programs, and public visibility campaigns that reflect the diversity of racial, gendered, and sexual identities within urban American Indian communities in the United States.

Chapter 4, "Gender and Racial Discrimination against Mixed-Race American Indian Two-Spirits," explores the impact of gender and racial discrimination as psychosocial factors that compound experiences of colonial trauma among MLGBTQ2S Natives. It proposes that Two-Spirit cultural dissolution opened a pathway for intergenerational and historical trauma that is re-actualized with each additional form of psychosocial risk.

Chapter 5, "Mixed-Race Identity, Cognitive Dissonance, and Public Health Among MLGBTQ2S," reviews the current literature in the field of public health in order to document the ways that MLGBTQ2S Native populations are often misunderstood, under researched, and mistakenly categorized as monoracial, non-Native individuals. If we are to have an active, inclusive, prevention-focused public health policy in this country, then there has to be a greater emphasis on mixed-race populations. Although these communities are growing by large numbers nationally, there is a glaring absence of foundational or baseline research measures for unpacking the cognitive dissonance that takes place among many individuals because of external (and sometime internal) identity ascription, a process that leads to a sense of marginalization or lack of belonging.

Chapter 6, "Sexual Violence and Transformative Ancestor Spirits," weighs sexual violence as a significant indicator of high-risk behavior and a psychosocial factor that increases the likelihood of contracting HIV as well as alcohol, drug, and mental health struggles. Chapter 6 also asserts that there is a movement among MLGBTQ2S Indigenous peoples, not just in the Bay Area but nationally, towards embracing ancestor spirits who were also Two-Spirit as role models for overcoming trauma and sexual violence. The participants in the book share the way that prayer to the ancestor spirits allows them to have an internal mechanism for participating in ceremony with their LGBT, Two-Spirit, mixed-blood ancestors.

Chapter 7, "Stress Coping in Urban Indian Kinship Networks," describes the efficacy of urban American Indian HIV/AIDS service organizations as well as other non-HIV-specific Indian cultural networks that offer a community-based approach to preventative healthcare. These projects seek to rebuild a sense of shared accountability, reciprocity, and kinship for community members, who for decades have felt isolated or excluded to varying degrees.

Chapter 8, "Two-Spirit Return: Intergenerational Healing and Cultural Leadership among Mixed-Race American Indians," proposes a two-year intervention to address the need for ongoing intergenerational healing between elders (over forty-five years of age) and youth (under forty-five years of age). This two-year intervention not only seeks to strengthen stress-coping mechanisms and systems of support for addressing colonial haunting and PTIS, but it also creates a specific leadership training program among MLGBTQ2S American Indians. These new leaders will have greater specific tribal knowledge, as well as an understanding of what I term traditional urban Indian cultural knowledge systems (TUICKS). As cultural leadership increases within the context of radical love and TUICKS, we will also witness a growth in Indigenous community organizing and the visibility of a community that together can collectively undo the notion that "Indian blood" is defined solely on the basis of biology, law, or phenotype, as opposed to cultural knowledge and community participation.

Indian Blood asks that we imagine a new way of defining group membership and, by extension, self-determination among Indigenous peoples in the United States and globally. In the same way that HIV/AIDS does not have to define as contaminated the lives and the blood of those who carry it, neither should mixed-race "blood" in a metaphoric, biological, or legal sense be used as a means for exclusion. A nation is stronger when all members are able to participate, especially those most at risk for ongoing colonial haunting and soul loss. We can strengthen health outcomes and policy by producing interventions that place the most vulnerable/marginalized among us at the center of our research. When we place the most marginalized at the center of our research, we are producing research as an act of justice, solidarity, and radical love within an Indigenous ceremonial context.

CHAPTER 2

Two-Spirit Cultural Dissolution

HIV and Healing among Mixed-Race American Indians

> You know there was, like, a mile of death up there,
> really serious death up there. So to me, like, when death is
> always open, all those old people are definitely gone.
> Those people are definitely gone.
>
> —Indian Blood focus group respondent

THE PSYCHOSOCIAL NEXUS OF RISK MODEL
AMONG MIXED-RACE AMERICAN INDIANS

This chapter builds on the findings of the pilot study "Indian Blood: Mixed-Race Gay Men, Transgender People, and HIV," which I conducted in partnership with the Native American AIDS Project (NAAP) in San Francisco from 2011 to 2012. Evidence to support the study of this particular population derives from national studies that indicate high HIV prevalence rates among mixed-race gay men (Valleroy, MacKellar, Karon, Rosen, McFarland, Shehan, and Douglas 2000) and disproportionate rates of infection among American Indians, who have the highest rate of interracial marriage among all U.S. ethnic groups (Lee and Edmonston 2005). Fifty participants of mixed ethnicity took part in four focus groups and completed demographic profile surveys to address Indigenous stress-coping mechanisms, mental health disparities, and HIV/AIDS risk among mixed-race American Indian gay men and transgender people. Data findings reveal high levels of racial and gender discrimination along with extremely high rates of reported sexual violence. Focus group analysis reveals a pattern of interconnected psychological and social risk factors for HIV/AIDS transmission within this population.

The Indian Blood Psychosocial Nexus of Risk (IBPN) model (figure 2.1) explains how six interrelated phenomena produce the conditions for higher risk behavior among MLGBTQ2S American Indians in the San Francisco Bay Area. Figure 2.1 graphically represents the shift from the traditional role of American Indian Two-Spirits as cultural and religious leaders within some tribal communities through a colonial process that stigmatizes those Indigenous peoples who identify as gay, lesbian, bisexual, or transgender in a contemporary context. I argue that as the spiritual, socioeconomic, and cultural significance of Two-Spirit individuals dissolved—through colonial contact with Europeans— MLGBTQ2S people experienced ruptures in their social and cultural support networks that under normal circumstances would serve as protective factors against external discrimination.[1] As discrimination against Two-Spirits has increased from contact to the present, a breakdown in traditional/community values, beliefs, and practices leads to detrimental experiences with intergenerational trauma and PTIS. These traumas within the context of the MLGBTQ2S experience are manifested through racial and gender discrimination, mixed-race cognitive dissonance, and sexual violence. If these traumas are left unaddressed by a traditional Two-Spirit cultural ethic of reciprocity then we can expect weak stress-coping mechanisms within urban Indian kinship networks. I also assert that the only way to heal from these traumas is through a return to a Two-Spirit cultural ethic of support, intergenerational mentoring, and ceremonial healing. Below I outline some of the ways that the IBPN model impacts MLGBTQ2S Natives.

POSSESSING AND DISPOSSESSING
THE TWO-SPIRIT SUBJECT

The process of Two-Spirit cultural dissolution for MLGBTQ2S American Indians has taken place over many centuries, during which the damage caused by colonization and ongoing settler colonialism has led to the dissolution of the cultural networks that supported Two-Spirit people (Jacobs, Lang, and Thomas 1997; Roscoe 1998; Giley 2006; and Morgensen 2011). The dissolution of Two-Spirit cultural practices is a direct result of the actions of religious missionaries and government officials who worked to erode, destroy, and reshape gender and sexual practices within Native communities throughout the Americas (Tinker 1993). Today many Indigenous communities have internalized and adopted some of these Western views of gender and sexuality. But there is a long history of Two-Spirit, third-gender, and fourth-gender military and religious

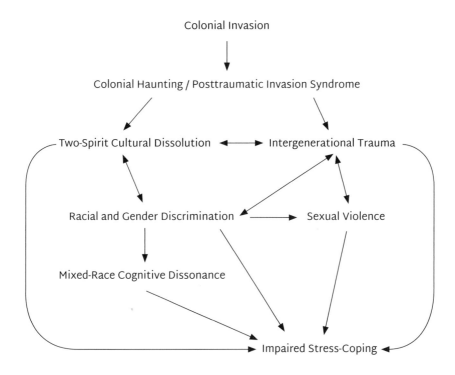

FIGURE 2.1. The Indian Blood psychosocial nexus of HIV risk model

leaders in tribes throughout the United States. The stigmas today attached to "non-normative" gender behavior were nonexistent in many tribal societies, as demonstrated by the story of Osh-Tisch (Finds Them and Kills Them), a traditional Crow *boté*, or third gender male. According to Will Roscoe, the *boté* "were experts in sewing and beading and considered the most efficient cooks in the tribe. According to one anthropologist, *boté* 'excelled women in butchering, tanning, and other domestic tasks'; another reported that their lodges were 'the largest and best appointed,' and that they were highly regarded for their charitable acts. Indeed by devoting themselves to women's work, which included everything connected with skins and their use in clothing, robes, moccasins, various accessories, and lodges (or tipis) free of interruption from childbearing and rearing, *boté* were in effect full-time craft specialists" (1998: 25–26).

This account demonstrates the range of social and cultural spaces that individuals whom we today call Two-Spirit or LGBTQ traditionally occupied in daily practices, without any sense of moral judgment from fellow tribal members. Today interdependent relationships and complex definitions of third- and fourth- gender identities and practices are absent. If we do witness these practices either through labor or ceremony, it is usually among those elders who still have knowledge, and marginal acceptance, of these precolonial practices of gender diversity. As the quote that opens this chapter suggests, what is left after all of "those old people are gone" is violence, lack of community cohesion, and weak or nonexistent kinship support networks. This transgender participant went on to state:

> You know, I've been to places where I've met people like myself on the reservation [who also attended boarding schools], but obviously [they] didn't like themselves enough because they didn't want to do nothing for themselves. But, um . . . I got beat up. I got the shit beat out of me so bad—you wouldn't even recognize me it was so bad. I got kicked in the face about twenty-five times by this guy with boots on. Just totally beat up on the reservation, nobody came to help, nobody helped me. . . . After leaving I got into a relationship but then I started using again. So it was like, you know what? You're gonna go back to the reservation and end up back where you were, go back downhill. Sobriety: that's why I came here. I needed to get the sobriety. And that was the main thing. Because what was up there for me was no longer [working].

Contemporary MLGBTQ2S American Indians like the respondent above are left without these supports because the elders who held the tribally specific knowledge have gone on and only Two-Spirit cultural dissolution and internalized Eurocentric values are left in their place. The values and beliefs of European missionaries and colonists led to the demise of the Two-Spirit identity in some communities. The acceptance of non-Native values and epistemologies has left many contemporary MLGBTQ2S people searching for community and cultural buffers to protect them in a world that sees them as aberrant both in mainstream and in internal ethnic group contexts. As Roscoe notes: "The values of European and American observers, however, led them to single out and denounce Crow customs regarding sexuality and gender. In 1889, when A. B. Holder reported observations of *boté* made during his assignment as a government doctor at the Crow agency, he concluded, 'Of all the many varieties of sexual perversion this, it seems to me, is the most debased that could be conceived of.' In this century, anthropologist Robert H. Lowie described Crow berdaches as 'pathological cases,' 'psychiatric cases,' 'abnormal,' 'anomalies,' 'perverts,' and 'inverts'" (Roscoe 1998: 26).

Traditional tribal gender and sexual systems that were accepting of many different individual expressions of gender and sexual identity only begin to erode as a result of conflicts over morality with colonists. The biological and the political were often merged with religious and military assaults on Native communities. All of this led to a process in which settler colonialism sought (and still seeks) to replace Indigenous ways of articulating gender and sexual identities and practices with European moral standards. As Morgensen argues, "in the Americas and specifically, the United States, the biopolitics of settler colonialism was constituted by the imposition of colonial heteropatriarchy and the hegemony of settler sexuality, which sought both the elimination of indigenous sexuality and its incorporation into settler sexual modernity" (2011: 34). The inherent contradiction of the imposition of settler sexuality narratives onto Indigenous peoples is that these narratives and interactions always sought to extinguish Indigenous sexual practices, while also studying and/or participating in Indigenous forms of sexuality.

Two-Spirit cultural dissolution is therefore a major aspect of what I term posttraumatic invasion syndrome (PTIS). After European invasion in the Americas, a process began in American Indian tribal societies that continues to produce painful memories of a history that is seldom told, but is very evident when we look at contemporary public health issues facing American Indians. These traumatic post-invasion experiences continue to threaten the well-being of MLGBTQ2S people, whose racial, gender, and sexual diversity make them one of the most marginalized groups in the United States. Because of their diversity and their perceived lack of authenticity, many contemporary MLGBTQ2S Natives—like those who participated in the Indian Blood study—are left isolated and looking for community support networks that will accept them for who they are regardless of their type of racial mixture, or whether they identify as queer, transgender, or some other category. MLGBTQ2S people also seek a shifting of policies that reduce their experiences to one aspect of their identities rather than speaking to each aspect of who they are as individuals and as a collective. This study aims to add to that search by asking how queer, Native-specific health organizations speak to the needs of multiracial clients.

One symptom of PTIS is the adoption of non-Native morals and values: when you change a people's cultural values and norms you change who they are as a people, often irrevocably. As Roscoe explains, prior to colonial invasion, every individual had a role and a purpose in tribal life—and the acceptance of Two-Spirit tribal members left the possibilities for contribution available to each individual fairly open. Among the Crow, for example, "if some individuals did not accept or were unsuited for the usual role assigned to their sex, they could still contribute to the community" (Roscoe 1998: 26–27). In the wake of colonization, with its narrower views of social normality, the options open to Two-Spirit individuals were severely curtailed.

Similarly, issues like same-sex marriage and culturally responsive public health programs remain challenges throughout most of the country. At the time of this writing, thirteen states, along with the District of Columbia and five Native American tribes (the Coquille, the Suquamish, the Little Traverse Bay Bands of Odawa Indians, the Pokagon Band of Potawatomi Indians, and the Lipay Nation of Santa Ysabel), had legalized same-sex marriage (Hotakainen 2013). On June 26, 2015, the Supreme Court, in a 5-4 vote, held that the Constitution guarantees the right to same-sex marriage. This ruling made same-sex marriage legal throughout the United States and dependent territories. But the decades-long battle for same-sex marriage did not end with the 2015 ruling. This legacy of this colonial policy continues to impact tribal nations, which can determine their own marriage laws. The fact that so many tribes have based their contemporary marriage laws on definitions of sex/gender is significant, considering that most tribes did not have such strict laws prior to the invasion. Such changes to Two-Spirit cultural values and practices through public health and legal policies have a direct impact on the spread of HIV/AIDS among MLG-BTQ2S Native Americans today.

POSTTRAUMATIC INVASION SYNDROME
AND MLGBTQ2S VULNERABILITIES

Posttraumatic invasion syndrome (PTIS) is defined here as the unnatural, geno-cidal disruption of entire Indigenous systems of cultural knowledge, practice, and self-determination through military, political, and religious exploitation and oppression, and the subconscious transference of invasion sickness and Indigenous nihilism as practiced and perpetrated against Native peoples to their own descendants from the early colonial period of the fifteenth century until the present colonial moment of the twenty-first century. PTIS is a sick-ness that has changed the epistemological and cosmological systems of many Indigenous peoples throughout the world. When we discuss for example LGBT persecution in Uganda, we must examine and measure the impact of PTIS on Ugandan government officials and everyday citizens. The same considerations

TWO-SPIRIT CULTURAL DISSOLUTION

must be taken into account when we look at MLGBTQ2S vulnerabilities for high-risk sexual behavior as a result of Two-Spirit cultural dissolution and subsequent, compounding psychosocial factors.

For American Indians, who make up the smallest percentage among U.S. racial groups, HIV/AIDS has steadily grown both on and off reservations. Irene Vernon, in her book *Killing Us Quietly: Native Americans and HIV/AIDS* (2001), explores how social concerns such as poverty, domestic violence, substance abuse, sexual molestation, and untreated mental illness have devastated Native gays and lesbians, along with Native youth and Native women, at alarming rates since 1984. According to Vernon, although use of alcohol and drugs is not itself a route of transmission for HIV, it plays a critical role in the AIDS epidemic: under the influence of substances, protective behaviors are often forgotten or ignored. Several HIV/AIDS-positive individuals within Vernon's book report that tribal communities not only deny that HIV/AIDS is a problem among American Indians but have also ostracized infected members. These actions create fear and mistrust, and therefore reluctance to obtain services. This social stigma also manifests itself in the context of risk behavior, as many displaced or marginal members of tribal communities who leave reservations and come to urban areas do not have the economic means, social networks, or access to vital services to receive adequate preventative services or adequate treatment post-seroconversion. Many of these urban Indians unfortunately become homeless, turn to prostitution, or become intravenous drug users, and many fall victim to all three of these social problems, all of which put them at greater risk for contracting HIV (Vernon 2001).

When issues of tribal displacement and relocation are combined with mixed-race identity, enrollment status, and queer identification, the result is greater levels of trauma and risk. The work of Karina Walters and her coinvestigators, in the article "Keeping Our Hearts from Touching the Ground: HIV/AIDS in American Indian and Alaska Native Women" (Walters, Evans-Campbell, Beltran, and Simoni 2011), suggests that the sustainability of American Indian communities is based on the health of the women within them, who have been central to the survival of so many communities throughout history, both pre- and post-invasion.

In traditional indigenous cosmologies, the feminine spirit is often regarded as that which sustains life. Even the earth, often referred to as "Mother Earth," is assigned a feminine identity who provides all that sustains human needs. Women and their bodies are representations of this life-sustaining force, and, in many indigenous cultures, women are regarded as agents of cultural and community preservation. As poetically articulated in the traditional Cheyenne proverb . . . a nation cannot be vanquished while the women remain strong enough in body and spirit to carry and protect not only physical but also cultural and spiritual survival. As such, survival of American Indian and Alaska Native (AIAN) cultures can be seen as integrally linked to Native women and this reality frames the need to protect their overall health and wellness, which is currently in a state of crisis. (S261–65)

I would argue that a similar assertion is true for Two-Spirit people. There have been attempts to fuse the past and the present as they relate to the practice of diverse gender and sexuality constructions, but I would suggest that we are still deeply entrenched in a decolonization project regarding both gender and sexuality. Until we can begin to move toward healing among all individuals within our communities—especially the most marginalized—we will continue to experience Two-Spirit cultural dissolution and a host of PTIS symptoms related to sexual violence, racial hybridity, and gender discrimination.

Ironically, even as Two-Spirit cultural dissolution creates divisions within Native communities, Two-Spirit identity/discourse is being put to use by non-Natives to appropriate a history associated with "authenticity" or "normativity" for their own same-sex relationships and political struggles. The use of precolonial Native and Indigenous religious, political, and cultural belief systems has long been available to non-Natives in ways that this same history is not readily accessible to the very people who descend from these traditions. These Native descendants have had these histories and practices taken away from them, only to be reused by non-Natives for their own political purposes. Morgensen (2011) notes that "U.S. queer projects define their integrity by appealing to the cultural status of an ethnic group or the legal status granted racial and national minorities, through 'racial analogy.' However, they have not asked how these normatively white and *non-Native* queer routes to 'race' play on indigeneity as a history or model of the authenticity they seek, while absenting Native people from the 'racial' queerness that secures citizenship" (91–92). Here, Morgensen argues convincingly that non-Native queer activists and scholars normalize their rights to "queer citizenship," based on racial entitlements attributed to Native peoples, whom they then deny "queer citizenship" on the basis of race. Thus, as queer citizenship is denied to MLGBTQ2S Natives by non-Native queers, racial citizenship is simultaneously denied them by many tribes and the U.S. government, both of which use blood quantum and other non-Native ideologies and practices to determine citizenship. In other words, not only is Two-Spirit cultural dissolution (including loss of acceptance for third- and fourth- gender people) taking place, but so is mixed-race exclusion, both as the result of internalizing Western ideas of what it means to be Native in the twenty-first century.

MIXED-RACE MARGINALIZATION AS
A TOOL OF QUEER/TRIBAL CITIZENSHIP

Queer and tribal citizenship are both based on notions of "authenticity" and "blood," and therefore many tribes have engaged in a practice of excluding both MLGBTQ2S and mixed-race American Indians as a way of "preserving" citizenship for the "real Indians" (Blu 1980, Forbes 1993, Sturm 2002, Garroutte 2002, Miles 2006, Jolivette 2007, Denetdale 2008, Barker 2012). The debates over marriage equality in the United States over the past decade, along with the repeal of DOMA (Defense of Marriage Act) in June 2013 and the Supreme Court ruling upholding the right to marry for same-sex couples in 2015, provide some basis for comparison between U.S. federal policy and those same policies as adopted by tribal governments. In her recent book *Native Acts: Law, Recognition, and Authenticity* (2012), Joanne Barker argues convincingly that disenrollment based on racial politics and gay marriage bans that mimic DOMA are each examples of internalized racism and homophobia within some Native communities; I contend that these developments are part of the cultural dissolution process for MLGBTQ2S. Barker points out that in the 2004 Cherokee same-sex marriage license refusal and the 2005 Diné Marriage Act represent colonial and heteronormative laws and policies adopted by American Indian tribes as a result of contact with Europeans during and throughout contact. As Barker states, "the Cherokee Nation and the Navajo Nation passed laws that mimicked the DOMA and state propositions to ban same-sex marriage rights and define marriage as being a union between a man and a woman. Invoking what had become code words for American patriotism, the tribes situated themselves as joining forces with 'the American people' to protect America against the threats that homosexuality and same-sex marriage posed for national security and social stability" (195).

In her analysis, Barker goes on to underscore the ways that non-Natives respond to the Cherokee and Navajo marriage policies, which they read as inconsistent with what they expect from Native American groups, whom they "logically" assume will be supportive of gay marriage because as "ethnic" minority groups, Natives are also discriminated against by the U.S. legal system. This response speaks to Morgensen's (2011) assertion that settler colonial sexuality is rooted in a queer citizenship that relies upon Native traditions while simultaneously erasing Native *ethnic bodies* from the discourse of queer citizenship. Where American Indian tribes themselves are concerned, after centuries of cultural dissolution and indoctrination about "blood," "citizenship," "Christian values," and "authenticity," why wouldn't they now hold many of the very same beliefs as the U.S. government? These examples of internalized oppression can clearly be traced to processes of social, political, economic, and cultural incorporation experienced through PTIS.

The history of mixed-race people in the United States is full of complexities, and some of the most pervasive racial tensions in this country have been attached to the separation of people of color and whites to prevent racial mixing. Anti-miscegenation laws in the United States made it illegal for Indigenous people and other people of color to marry whites in many parts of the country up until 1967, when the Supreme Court repealed the anti-miscegenation laws that still existed in seventeen states (Dominguez 1993, Daniel 2001, Johnson 2003).

Research on mixed-race populations has focused on the psychological and mental impacts of being mixed-race, and especially of being biracial. Early eugenics research suggested that the offspring of these interracial unions would produce the worst type of individual (Darwin 1859, Galton 1869, Davenport 1929, Stonequist 1937). This mixed-race individual, these theorists argued, would suffer from confusion and would not effectively belong to, nor be able to integrate into, any of their ancestral communities. Subsequent research, often conducted by multiracial people, has focused on trying to celebrate and reclaim the rights of mixed-race people to identify with every aspect of their identity, emphasizing identity development, self-esteem, and cultural competence (Root 1992, 1995; Penn 1998; Ifekwunigwe 2004). Still, current research is only beginning to examine the impact of counting people of mixed-race identity as more than one race (Dacosta 2007, Odell-Korgen 2010, Wijeyesinghe and Jackson 2012). Until 2000, the U.S. Census did not allow people to choose two or more races or a multiracial category. Between 2000, when that policy changed, and 2010, the self-identified multiracial population has grown by more than 35 percent; according to the 2010 census and subsequent data collected in 2012 multiracial people under the age of eighteen are the fastest-growing youth demographic in the state of California.

The Census Board's decision to include a "two or more races" category incited tremendous debate within communities of color, as valuable resources are attached to the results of each federal census. Backlash against the "multiracial census movement" caused a resurfacing of older issues about community loyalties for mixed-race individuals within communities of color. Public consideration of these tensions however has tended to focus primarily on relationships between whites and people of color as opposed to relationships among people of color (Wilson 1993) or to the marginalization experienced by mixed-race people who have parents from two minority backgrounds. Today, we know that mixed-race youth are the fastest-growing youth demographic not only in California but also in many parts of the United States (U.S. Census 2000). We know that mixed-race youth are experiencing multiple forms of marginalization within mainstream society and within Indigenous people of color communities.

Much of the current public health research looking at experiences of racial discrimination fails to address issues that specifically impact people of mixed descent, in part because the inclusion of the "two or more races" category is relatively recent. There is still no data representing how mixed-race people deal with discrimination, whether in school, employment, labor, or health. Most of the research in this area assumes that all mixed-race people have at least one white parent and therefore that these individuals have more privilege than monoracial individuals of color. These assumptions have led to stagnant research agendas, with little attention given to the salience of racial hybridity in health outcomes for underserved populations. This chapter argues that mixed-race identity intersects with gender and sexuality to produce particular life experiences and health risks unique to mixed-race American Indian people who also identity as LGBT, queer, or Two-Spirit.

The quote that opens this chapter not only speaks to the declining presence of traditional values, given that elders are "gone," but it also reveals the ways that violence within tribal contexts has become endemic, as a result of colonial perspectives that shift the role of Two-Spirits from one of importance to one of deviance, marking them as unworthy of community acceptance or protection. The literal and symbolic death of "the old ways" leaves MLGBTQ2S without an effective kinship network of community support.

Many of the respondents express their difficulty in finding a community of support in the urban environment. They feel that without organizations like NAAP that can serve as surrogate kinship support networks, they will experience levels of exclusion and violence similar to those they experienced within rural, reservation settings where seemingly all of the elders who held traditional knowledge have died, leaving new—colonial and non-Indigenous— views in their place. As one respondent explained,

It felt like . . . it almost felt like just because we're Indian and we don't hang
out or things like that but I mean . . . I always wanted to be friends with Indians, but they always seemed kinda like I was . . . I felt like not really Indian
because I was raised by white people so it was kind of . . . I was always kind
of shy and I didn't identify with Indian issues. But um . . . it was when I came
to NAAP that I was able to find out about BAAITS and all these wonderful
organizations that have to do with American Indian people. So I learned how
to bead, and like all these wonderful things—like, I'd been wanting to experience all these wonderful things for many years and I never knew that I could
because I just never thought about it.

It is important to understand the difficulty that people of mixed-race backgrounds experience throughout their lifetimes. In the case of mixed-race American Indians, these experiences of discrimination and historical trauma are
compounded by the oppression directed towards American Indians, who are
often miscategorized racially or seen as a small population with no statistical
relevance to public health research. Several participant comments demonstrate
how MLGBTQ2S cultural dissolution, coupled with intergenerational trauma
within the family sphere, impacted their use of drugs and alcohol, thereby
producing high-risk sexual behavior.

I grew up by myself and um, a lot of ducking and dodging, you know, a lot
of—it was just a constant. A constant life, you know, so um . . . and my family didn't know how to deal with it 'cause my mother was working all of the
time, she didn't know what was going on, and I don't know, I was drunk a lot
too, you know. I started smoking cigarettes, I learned how to inhale when
I was about five or six years old and I liked it. I was smoking and my sister
would let me smoke. By the time I turned thirteen, my mother allowed me
to smoke cigarettes, she allowed me to smoke weed, she allowed me to do
speed—she let me do whatever I wanted. As long as I did what I was supposed to do, you know.

Another respondent's comment about drugs and alcohol within the context
of dating and relationships underscores the how family trauma and substance
abuse, passed from one generation to the next, cause a soul wound, and neces-
sitate the development of a cultural leadership and healing model to address
Two-Spirit cultural dissolution.[2]

Umm . . . I've been in two relationships. And both of them were not good. The first one, I was fifteen, and the guy was, like, ten years older than me, and he just wanted me because I was young, so, um . . . it was bad because, you know, he was supplying me with, you know, alcohol and, giving me drugs and stuff like that, so . . . that's how that relationship went. And then there was another one, and that one . . . was like, you know, I got into the relationship but I didn't want to be in it. Because, you know, I was already addicted to, you know, drugs and drinking alcohol and stuff, and, you know, I didn't—I wanted the drugs and alcohol more than I wanted that person, you know . . .

These passages demonstrate the interconnected nature of Two-Spirit cultural dissolution with alcohol, drug abuse, and mental health disparities within mixed-blood American Indian communities. Among study participants, 50 percent reported having had experiences with racial discrimination within a six-month period; when measured over a twelve-month period, the figure rises to 58 percent. In the same twelve-month time period, 56 percent reported having experienced sexual violence. The high prevalence of both racial discrimination and, sexual violence strongly indicates the need for an intervention to heal and restore cultural practices that strengthen protective factors against the transmission of HIV.

To effectively address discrimination experienced by mixed-race American Indians there must be a return to Two-Spirit traditional values and ceremonial practices that are tribally specific as well as community driven. As we have seen, studies conducted on the history, importance, and leadership roles played by Two-Spirits in tribal societies reveal a pattern of not only acceptance, but often document a place of reverence for Two-Spirits within their tribal nations (Jacobs, Thomas, and Lang 1997, Roscoe 1998, Giley 2006).

When Two-Spirit cultural dissolution is coupled with mixed-race cognitive dissonance, it leads to mental stress and the potential for greater high-risk behavior. Consider the following dilemma faced by one of the study participants within his own home when hybridity became a challenge for him as a mixed-blood Native person:

Well I think that um . . . I think the racial aspect came to me relatively early because, like I said, I grew up in the '70s. So when I was a little kid . . . AIM was really getting under way in Oklahoma . . . and my father was involved with AIM for, like, a short while. Um . . . and that actually caused a lot of friction at home because [of] my mother being white. Then my father would always come home and complain and talk about, you know, "white people this" and "white people that." And everything and so . . . I think from a very young age I started learning the difference between who was Native and who was white. And I guess also very young I learned the word "half-breed" was not a catchy tune. It was an insult designed specifically for people that are mixed. And um . . . and I can't tell you how much it sticks in my craw when somebody says, "Oh, so you're a half-breed." It kills me every time. I just hate it.

This respondent's experience with racial discrimination in his own household reveals the ways in which mixed-race cognitive dissonance can compound one's risk for HIV transmission in the absence of a supportive home environment free from intergenerational trauma and sexual violence. Other participant responses suggest that a chaotic home environment and weak kinship support networks normalize sexual violence and molestation, which might explain why some participants engage in high-risk sexual behavior as adults.

I grew up on the Navajo Indian Reservation. I was born in the early '60s and I fell into alcohol and drugs. My parents, um, they owned a bar and my father—my mother was my father's third wife. So I was born a [booze] baby, I was expected to die. I think I was a preemie. I had a lot of problems; you know a lot of [them]. I used to be a runt and, um, I got teased a lot. I got picked on all the way back. From the beginning, maybe one or two [years old] and I knew when the drinking was going around, I participated in the drinking. I grew up with an adult mind. And I talked. A lot of things when you talk, there are a few things that go on in the house, you know, to other people that don't live there, you know, it's an issue—but it was a party house. A lot of drinking, a lot of drugs, a lot of abuse—physical, verbal, mental, and spiritual. Um, by the time I was like four years old, some of the older guys, you know, they would try to molest me, but each and every time that they ever did, I did it consensually. I knew that if I was going to say something, then I was talking too much or there always some kind of an issue going on around me. And when I think I was around three-and-a-half, four years old, my father used to sell drugs and of course you know my parents, they would know that it's wrong. They wouldn't want it to happen, but . . . And I got abused, you know, from the way he had to set an example before all of my cousins, my relations. Everybody would come around the house. I'd get teased all the way to school, all the way during school, all the way back, it was just always constantly conflict with everyone. So more or less I grew up on my own.

The above understanding of "consent" demonstrates the extreme degree to which intergenerational trauma and PTIS has allowed for the reproduction of social and psychological abuse within the MLGBTQ2S population. Research on the experiences of mixed-race people, particularly as it relates to health and wellness, is scant or almost nonexistent. Because studies of the risk factors for HIV among mixed-race American Indian men and mixed-race transgender people is also woefully limited, the data collected during the pilot phase of this study attempts to bring greater visibility to the intersections between mixed-race identity, HIV, public health, and healing.

As much as this research is about documenting risk factors for HIV transmission, such as racial discrimination, sexual violence, and substance abuse, the book is also an attempt to thoroughly document through empirical and qualitative data, the lived experiences of racially mixed, queer American Indians. This chapter further reveals how Two Spirit cultural dissolution as a result of colonial invasion is a key cause of intergenerational trauma within MLGBTQ2S American Indian communities. If we are to reduce risk for HIV transmission and improve healing within the mixed-race American Indian community then we must return to Native values and beliefs that support and respect the participation of MLGBTQ2S people within the broader American Indian community.

Data from the original pilot study in 2012 suggests that intergenerational gaps in cultural knowledge and community participation contribute significantly to increased behavioral risk among MLGBTQ2S people. One goal of this book is to formulate an intergenerational healing and cultural leadership (IHCL) model, detailed in chapter 8, that will not only provide empirical data, but also address gaps in ethnic-specific, community-based networks of support among MLGBTQ2S Natives. This intervention, by its design, seeks to restore the cultural networks of support that were once provided by Two-Spirit leaders in American Indian communities. The goal of the IHCL model is to produce effective urban Indian kinship networks of support and healing between different generations of mixed-blood American Indians. If successful, this model will provide the community with another method to combat intergenerational trauma and Two-Spirit cultural dissolution while simultaneously reducing HIV risk among MLGBTQ2S American Indians.

Reducing rates of HIV risk among MLGBTQ2S Natives and introducing the IHCL model is particularly significant because, despite the relatively low overall number of new cases of HIV infection among American Indians nationally, American Indian health disparities may be missed in Census data, due to the growing number of individuals who identify with two or more races. We must make a conscientious effort to disaggregate these statistics to better understand the data as they relate to American Indian and Alaska Natives of mixed descent. According to Walters, Evans-Campbell, Beltran, and Simoni (2011), American Indians and Alaska Natives diagnosed with AIDS had shorter survival times than whites, Asians and Pacific Islanders, multiracial people, and Hispanics.[3]

> Though the number of AIDS cases among AIANs reported by the Centers for Disease Control (CDC) accounts for less than 1 percent of the total in the United States, this statistic fails to represent the actual impact on AIAN communities. Prior to the breaking-out of multiple race and Native Hawaiian/Pacific Islanders as categories of surveillance, AIANs ranked third in rate of diagnoses behind African Americans and Hispanics (CDC 2008). Since the changes to race/ethnic surveillance data, AIAN now rank fifth in diagnoses behind African Americans, Hispanic/Latinos, Native Hawaiian/Pacific Islanders, and persons identifying as multiple races; however, the report advises caution when interpreting this data as the number of Native Hawaiian/Pacific Islanders is small and consequently unstable. Further complicating this data is the reality that Native Hawaiians/Pacific Islanders are Indigenous peoples and share similar historical and contemporary experiences related to colonization, ongoing discrimination, and persistent health disparities (S261–65).

The fact that infection rates are increasing rapidly among this population, and that people who identify as multiracial have high rates of AIDS diagnosis, demonstrates that there may indeed be serious underreporting of HIV/AIDS incidence rates among people of American Indian descent. In order to fully bring a sense of healing to this community, it is necessary that we unpack the identity categories constructed by the West and internalized by Natives and non-Natives alike. Healing takes many generations and multiple forms of intervention.

As we proceed with our discussion of MLGBTQ2S identity and the correlations between gender, race, and sexuality in the face of colonial haunting and HIV, we will need to carefully outline a shift in policy, education, and public discourse that creates a more fluid space for people to be their full selves in every social space that they occupy. Decolonizing gender, sexuality, and mixed-race identity will require an understanding of the ways that settler colonialism, coupled with Two-Spirit cultural dissolution and PTIS, create the conditions for psychosocial risks to be created, maintained, and transformed by Natives and non-Natives. In this co-constitutive process of decolonization, we can create new paradigms that respect the self-determination of MLGBTQ2S communities that have long suffered and awaited their healing moment.

CHAPTER 3

Historical and Intergenerational Trauma and Radical Love

I started smoking cigarettes, I learned how to inhale,
when I was about five or six years old, and I liked it. I was
smoking and my sister would let me smoke. By the time I
turned thirteen, my mother allowed me to smoke cigarettes,
she allowed me to smoke weed, she allowed me to do speed,
she let me do whatever I wanted. As long as I did
what I was supposed to do, you know.

—Indian Blood focus group respondent

AMERICAN INDIAN AND INDIGENOUS PEOPLES CONTINUE TO SUFFER
from various inequities in health, education, and employment. The U.S. government's policies from the beginning of contact with Native peoples have included
political and economic incorporation processes that have produced unimagina-
ble traumas that are both legally embedded and "morally" sanctioned (Cornell
1990, Tinker 1993). These historical traumas are culturally, economically, and
spiritually transferred from one generation to the next. The resulting intergenerational traumas are not only endemic within Native communities, they
are also central to U.S polices of control, paternalism, and global imperialism.

Decolonizing gender and sexuality does not imply a return to a precolonial
imaginary. Rather, to decolonize gender and sexuality within the context of
trauma requires a releasing of each of the epistemological narratives that limit
the definitions of what it means to be Native, mixed-race, Two-Spirit, and/or
queer. Decolonization cannot exist without some degree of what I term radical
love. Radical love is ultimately a theory of communal responsibility, trust, and
vulnerability. The challenge in moving toward healing within MLGBTQ2S communities is to produce effective mechanisms of trust so that queer, mixed-race,
Native peoples can experience vulnerability on their own terms and with their

47

own people. For MLGBTQ2S Natives to allow themselves to become vulnerable, after remembered centuries of traumatic experience, requires a willingness to trust others, to forgive the self, and even to forgive those who commit acts of violence and abuse. Elsewhere, I've defined radical love as follows:

> Radical love is about being vulnerable. It is about being unafraid to speak out about issues that may not have a direct impact on us on a daily basis. Radical love is about caring enough to admit when we are wrong and to admit to mistakes. Radical love should ask how the work in which we are engaged helps to build respectful relationships between ourselves and others involved in social justice movements. Radical love asks if we are each being responsible in fulfilling our individual roles and obligations to the other participants in the struggle for social justice and human rights. Finally, radical love in critical mixed race studies means asking ourselves if what we are contributing is giving back to the community and if it is strengthening the relationships of all of those involved in the process. Is what is being shared adding to the growth of the community and is this sharing reciprocal? Is what we are working toward leading to a more peaceful and equitable society? (Jolivette 2012: n.p.)

In order to begin a process of decolonization that can effectively incorporate radical love and address intergenerational trauma, we must first distinguish between posttraumatic stress disorder (PTSD) and posttraumatic invasion syndrome (PTIS). Posttraumatic stress disorder (PTSD) has been passed from generation to generation, clan group to clan group, and family to family across Native North America. Maria Yellow Horse Brave Heart (2003) cites the following as potential outcomes of PTSD: identifying with the dead, depression, psychic numbing, hypervigilance, fixation to trauma, suicidal ideation and gestures, survivor guilt, loyalty to ancestral suffering, low self-esteem, anger distortion, revictimization by people in authority, mental illness, fear of authority and intimacy, domestic and lateral violence, inability to assess risk, and reenactments of abuse in disguised form. Posttraumatic invasion syndrome (PTIS) stems from the specific responses of Indigenous peoples to ongoing settler violence and is distinct from PTSD in identifying invasion as a lifelong experience that often begins at birth and when unaddressed does more than create stress: it destabilizes families and entire tribal communities. The manifestations of PTSD and PTIS from historical traumas lead to intergenerational and cyclical patterns of what I term *spirit-traumas*. Spirit-traumas cause severe emotional and cultural blockages that make it difficult if not impossible to regain a sense of individual and group autonomy, self-determination, and spiritual resiliency in the face of colonial haunting, out of fear of reexperiencing painful memories and traumas either from childhood or ancestors. Many of the participants I spoke with throughout the course of my research with NAAP provide testimony that speaks to the prevalence of ongoing colonial traumas and spirit-traumas that weaken their stress-coping mechanisms when it comes to changing high-risk social, psychological, and sexual behaviors.

Scholars for more than a decade have examined intergenerational trauma as a factor in health outcomes. Many studies on trauma suggest that stress-coping mechanisms and culturally appropriate health services can mitigate some of the risk factors produced by intergenerational trauma. I assert that radical love and vulnerability may be one of the most effective coping mechanisms for combating trauma between generations. Silence in Native communities is one of the leading factors in the current spread of the HIV virus. The tension between Native and Western science and how best to address issues of PTSD and other health disparities is of paramount importance for the future sustainability of Indigenous communities in North America. According to Colorado (1988), "the purpose of aboriginal science is to understand WHY or ultimate causality. For Western science the purpose is to describe HOW or the immediate causality." The divergence in epistemological approaches between Native and Western science is important for addressing historical trauma because Western science assumes that the past is the past and that individuals are capable of responding to their own current situations. Take for example the fact that most psychotherapy sessions are done one-on-one with a therapist who is initially at least a stranger. This context is not conducive for being vulnerable, placing trust, or achieving healing. Ultimately the difference between Western and Native sciences lies in a quest for immediate and short-term solutions versus long-term and ongoing solutions—"curing" versus healing. While there are schools of psychotherapy, such as relational and feminist approaches, that examine the relationship between vulnerability, trust, intimacy, and healing, many psychotherapy modalities still focus on individual versus collective healing.

The participants in the Indian Blood study were able to achieve high levels of vulnerability and honesty with one another, despite years of experiencing mental, physical, and sexual violence both from members of their own communities and from outsiders. Still, residual feelings of vulnerability among the participants suggest the need for additional intervention work to address ongoing spirit-traumas. Spirit-traumas prevent many MLGBTQ2S Natives from integrating their physical and mental health issues into a single coherent stress-

TABLE 3.1. Theoretical Models for Native and Western Science

	Native Science	Western Science
Purpose	To understand why, or the ultimate causality	To describe how, or the immediate causality
Methods	Talking with elders, prayer, fasting, and traditional ceremonies	Measuring, breaking things down to their smallest parts, analyzing data
Outcome measures	Balance within and with the natural world.	A report of findings and data analysis
Subjective approach	The scientist or researcher puts himself or herself into the study	The scientist or researcher separates himself or herself and his or her feelings from the study
Spiritual approach	Spirituality is in everything and everything is interconnected	Religion is separate from science
Locus of control	Community	Outside experts

Adapted from Colorado 1988.

coping or healing mechanism. Pervasive and ongoing psychological violence in Indian Country prevents many individuals from seeking help, especially within the context of colonial haunting in their own communities and Native environments. For many MLGBTQ2S American Indians, seeking support within their own communities is tremendously difficult because historical trauma produces a unique form of internalized ecological-colonialism that negates the full experience of mixed-race, LGBTQ, and Two-Spirit people within their own nations.

While *Indian Blood* specifically examines urban mixed-race Indians, it also considers the experiences of MLGBTQ2S American Indians who grow up in rural and reservation settings. Colorado's 1988 study of Aboriginal (Native) and Western approaches to science (see Table 3.1) reveals how disconnection between these modes is central problem in addressing issues of decolonization related to gender, sexuality, and mixed-race identity for Native peoples living with or at high risk for HIV transmission.

The most striking differences between Western and Native approaches to understanding historical and intergenerational trauma relate to purpose and methodology. Transmission of historical trauma, like transmission of HIV, cannot be prevented without examining ultimate causality nor without practicing traditional methods specific to Indigenous ways of knowing and achieving well-being. Numerous scholars are producing important work that investigates the correlations between historical trauma and health disparities among Indigenous peoples (Walters and Simoni 2002; Walters, Simoni, and Evans-Campbell 2002).

HISTORICAL TRAUMA AND HEALTH DISPARITIES AMONG INDIGENOUS PEOPLES

Historical trauma continues to produce health disparities because certain behaviors, policies, and practices remain invisible and unchanged within U.S. government policy. That is to say that many survivors of historical trauma do not want to remember the events of the past, though it is in that remembering that healing can actually begin. Remembering traumatic events can be at once both retriggering and healing. When an individual remembers what has taken place to him or her or to ancestors, it can open up the possibility for reexperiencing past traumas and create anxieties that in turn lead to behaviors associated with higher risk of HIV transmission. According to Duran and Duran (1995), "if these traumas are not resolved in the lifetime of the person suffering such upheaval, it is unthinkable that the person will not fall into some type of dysfunctional behavior that will then become the learning environment for their children. . . . This dysfunction and oppression have been internalized to such a degree that the oppressed members of the family seemingly want to continue to be oppressed or abused" (35). The shift away from communal to individual approaches for healing not only weakens stress- and trauma-coping mechanisms, but it also disrupts tribal cultural environments. As Duran and Duran explain, "Native American people were able to have a centered awareness that was fluid and nonstatic. [This] centered awareness allowed for a harmonious attitude toward the world, as exemplified by a tribal collective way of life versus an individualistic approach" (45). Destabilizing tribal collective ways of life leads to environmental racism and oppression, which are key factors in the transmission of HIV/AIDS; like other health disparities among vulnerable populations, HIV/AIDS infection rates are produced by social and legal policies, not merely biological predispositions.

Colonization may not be the only factor in ongoing health disparities facing American Indians, but it is one of the most salient contributing factors in the spread of physical disease and mental illness, as well as massive rates of

Native mortality. As we have seen, PTIS as an ongoing settler colonial experience contributes to an increase in current health disparities facing American Indian communities in the United States. According to David Jones (2006) in "The Persistence of American Indian Health Disparities":

> Mortality increased soon after the arrival of Christopher Columbus, and it quickly reached catastrophic proportions. Estimates of precontact American populations vary between 8 and 112 million (2 to 12 million for North America), and estimates of total mortality range from 7 to 100 million. Whatever the exact numbers, the mortality was unprecedented and overwhelming. Every new encounter brought new epidemics. Smallpox, measles, influenza, and malaria (and possibly hepatitis, plague, chickenpox, and diphtheria) spread into Mexico and Peru during the sixteenth century, New France and New England during the seventeenth century, and throughout North America and the Pacific islands during the eighteenth and nineteenth centuries. Populations often decreased by more than 90 percent during the first century after contact (2124).

In almost every one of the leading causes of death within the United States, American Indians experience disproportionate rates of mortality when compared with the general population, as a result of economics and of differences in methods of prevention, treatment, and medical adherence.[1] As I've argued throughout this chapter, high levels of distrust of Western medical institutions as a result of colonization and scientific abuses in Indigenous communities—ranging from forced sterilization to fraudulent clinical trials to studies that map Native peoples' DNA—make it difficult for American Indians to engage with Western medicine. Health insurance has also been a key indicator for long-term health and wellness as well as for measuring the effectiveness of preventative medicine in prolonging group life expectancy. According to the 2010 census, 29 percent of American Indians were living without life insurance. Despite the passage of the Affordable Care Act, the number of uninsured people in Native communities still sits at nearly 30 percent, in large part because of mistrust of U.S. programs that historically only deepened suffering in these communities (Vestal 2013). Issues such as access to effective health services, poverty, and unemployment also exacerbate intergenerational trauma and in turn fuel high-risk behavior. Thirty-Four percent of Indian Blood study participants were unemployed, retired, homeless, disabled, or living on SSI. Social and economic living conditions for American Indians have not improved much over the past five centuries. The ongoing and renewed colonial interest in Native land, resources, and capital has not subsided since first contact. The often-cited "Indian problem" persists into the twenty-first century: as more and more people self-identify as Native, there is a simultaneous struggle to preserve Indigenous languages, knowledge systems, ceremonies, and health practices.

Urbanization and by extension potential access to larger, better equipped urban hospitals and medical centers does not necessarily improve the lives of Native peoples because there are structural inequalities in the access and delivery mechanisms that are supposed to provide adequate preventative health care. Further, because more than 67 percent of Native people live in urban areas and away from their reservations, many cannot access Indian Health Services (IHS). Over the years, IHS has had a troubled relationship with American Indians and Alaska Natives in terms of its ability to effectively support their health needs. When IHS was initially instituted in 1955, the organization had an enormous task ahead: how to address nearly five centuries of health disparities (Jones 2006). Because IHS is run by the federal government there have been gaps in its provision of culturally appropriate health care services for Natives, exacerbated by "persistent anxiety and mistrust stemming from the often embattled relations between Native nations and the U.S. government" (Ditewig-Morris, Blue, and Folsom 2011). Statistics reveal startling correlations between historical trauma, poverty, and health disparities that continue to receive little to no attention in mainstream media: "Some researchers assert that historical influences are direct contributors to the current social and health problems found in American Indian populations. They link high rates of suicide, substance abuse, mental illness, domestic violence and other social ills to unresolved grief" (Morris, Blue, and Folsom 2011). This unresolved grief weighs on the emotional stability and physical capacity of many American Indians, especially those who are also racially mixed, because they are deeply challenged by others who often do not recognize them as "authentic" Natives (Barker 2012).

Grief related to spirit-traumas and internalized ecological-colonialism must be addressed in order to combat the increasing numbers of Native people living with HIV/AIDS. When taken together as a group, American Indians/Alaska Natives and Native Hawaiians have the third- and fourth- highest rates of new HIV infections respectively (Ditewig-Morris, Blue, and Folsom 2011). Within groups living with AIDS, American Indians and Alaska Natives have the shortest survival rate following diagnosis, followed by Native Hawaiians (Ditewig-Morris, Blue, and Folsom 2011).

Many of the MLGBTQ2S American Indians I spoke with cited difficulty in navigating the many possible vehicles for health care service, especially as they transitioned from rural or reservation living to larger urban centers in San Francisco and Oakland. According to a 2008 National Alliance of State and Territorial AIDS Directors (NASTAD) technical assistance report, there are multiple complex and overlapping issues to consider in meeting the needs of Native people at risk for or already living with HIV or AIDS. Perhaps most difficult is navigating the bureaucracy required to obtain health insurance and gain access to the health services necessary to have a measureable impact on HIV prevention and life-expectancy rates for American Indians and Alaska Natives.

It is my contention that unaddressed historical trauma, coupled with bureaucratic barriers to health care access, leaves many MLGBTQ2S American Indians at a loss as to how to find adequate services, networks of support, and healing. The recent work of Native scholars offers some hope in dealing with historical trauma and some possible indicators for how to reduce barriers to health care access.

Moving forward in the work of reducing the transmission of HIV/AIDS requires more recognition of historical and intergenerational trauma as co-constitutive social phenomena that increase risk for seroconversion. These two forms of trauma require the same treatment as other forms of genocide. Recognizing historical and intergenerational trauma as acts of genocide will also require a turn to the United Nations, specifically to the UN Declaration on the Rights of Indigenous Peoples, to address three key aspects of Indigenous colonial haunting: law, including self-determination, sovereignty, and reciprocity; land, including religion, ceremony, kinship, and love; and language, including culture, knowledge, education, and history. Bringing formal, international, legal attention to HIV/AIDS in Indigenous communities as a form of genocide pulls away the mask of colonial haunting, which will otherwise continue to incite fear, isolation, and high-risk behaviors associated with PTSD and spirit-trauma across Indian Country.

INTERGENERATIONAL TRAUMA AS A COLONIAL HAUNTING AND GENOCIDAL PRACTICE

When one study participant was asked if HIV/AIDS had had any effect on his sexual practices and behaviors, he replied, "It scared me. [It has] taken people I've known. I try to be careful. Sometimes you suspend responsible thought and action though." This response demonstrates how intergenerational trauma as a colonial haunting produces genocidal practices. This person also described his family environment when he was growing up as dysfunctional, citing the fact that the family moved around a lot. This MLGBTQ2S person is also homeless and states that his sources of social support are "kind of flimsy right now: some social agencies, some friends . . . It's rough right now." Trauma reproduces itself generation after generation because there has been no interruption of patterns of abusive, psychological violence, nor any concentration on restoring cultural buffers and social support networks: like this respondent, many MLGBTQ2S American Indians have "flimsy" support networks. In a follow-up question related to how participants deal with stress, this respondent said, "Unfortunately, [I] usually drink."

In their coauthored essay, "Reconceptualizing Native Women's Health: An 'Indigenist' Stress-Coping Model" (2002), Karina Walters and Jane Simoni argue that intergenerational trauma or cumulative trauma produces high rates of posttraumatic stress disorder and other forms of psychological distress, most likely due to high rates of violence. Walters and Simoni further posit that historical trauma in particular (e.g., boarding school exposure, coercive migration, and non-Native custodial care placements) should also factor into our understanding of poor health outcomes for Native people. The authors offer the "Indigenist" stress-coping model as a framework for understanding the causal relationships between historical trauma, intergenerational trauma, and cultural buffers in assessing health risks and outcomes for Native women. This model advocates identifying ways to thoroughly integrate "social, psychological, and cultural reasoning about discrimination and other forms of trauma as determinants of health" (Walters and Simoni 2002: 520–24).

Walters and Simoni's model provides a critical pathway for understanding the uniqueness of stress-coping mechanisms utilized by Indigenous peoples. *Indian Blood* aims to understand and use the Indigenist stress-coping mechanism developed by Walters and Simoni to understand how MLGBTQ2S Natives deal with stress in their live as a result of ongoing colonial stigmas. Colonial haunting for example, produces limits and conditions on the possibility of living a full and complete life, one free of social stigmas as a result of experiences with unresolved grief, mourning, and multiple forms of physical displacement, from removal to relocation to marginal housing or homelessness. The indigenist stress-coping model provides sociocultural and economic reasoning as opposed to pathological explanations for the epidemiological overrepresentation of American Indian communities in the HIV/AIDS epidemic. Organizations that are ethnic-specific, like NAAP, provide fundamentally important tools for combating historical trauma, discrimination (in terms of race, gender, and sexuality, among others), and traumatic life events such as physical and sexual assaults. As noted in the previous chapter, more than half of the Indian Blood study participants reported having experienced sexual assault, ranging from molestation and incest to rape. The stigmas associated with being MLGBTQ2S coupled with intergenerational trauma create the conditions for multiple forms of societal marginalization that only increase rates of HIV transmission within this demographic, but also isolate those who are already HIV positive.

As one respondent said, "I'm HIV positive. Sometimes I feel this limits my dating pool to gay positives. I tend to feel gay positives are either really mature or totally fucked up. I wish there was more middle ground." This absence of middle ground is true for many MLGBTQ2S who are working on issues of shame, vulnerability, and healing. Organizations like NAAP are important if there is to be a systematic and continuous response to HIV/AIDS in Native communities. However, with high levels of competition for resources, as discussed earlier, organizations like NAAP are not able to sustain themselves and many successful ethnic-specific organizations end up closing their doors, as NAAP did. The level of care and support that an individual needs after living with intergenerational trauma for many years is not easily understood by most mainstream health care facilities. One respondent, when asked why they chose NAAP, said, "The reason I chose NAAP is because of how much they all care about everyone." Another respondent who identifies as transgender stated that "they have good support groups and prevention steps at NAAP." She went on to say that her gender identity plays an important role in where she chooses to obtain services because, "I'm a Native transgender [woman] and my risks for getting HIV are higher." This woman, who has always identified as female, recognizes how her multiple identities as Native, transgender, and mixed-blood impact her risk for acquiring HIV, so she intentionally chose to seek services at an ethnic-specific organization that could help her deal with all of the issues associated with intergenerational trauma and genocide.

Over 80 percent of participants stated that they have ways of dealing with discrimination and stress. This high number initially came as a surprise to me. As I thought more carefully about the impact of intergenerational trauma, I realized that it was because in the context of NAAP the participants were able to be vulnerable, to move forward with their lives and seek out services. However, such people represent a small percentage of the population that needs help. It also became clear that without NAAP—and particularly its male, female, and transgender talking circles—many participants would have no other place to turn for support in dealing with stress and discrimination. Ethnic-specific organizations like NAAP successfully reduce HIV risk factors such as intergenerational trauma for MLGBTQ2S Natives in ways that mainstream health organizations and facilities cannot, because NAAP and similar organizations provide cultural toolkits that reduce barriers to practicing safer sex and other healthy social behaviors. Now that NAAP's doors are closed, I often wonder what has become of some of the MLGBTQ2S people that I got to know and learn from over the course of this study.

RADICAL LOVE AND MLGBTQ2S HEALTH
AND CULTURAL RECOVERY

Radical love, which organizations like NAAP and BAAITS are able to offer their communities, needs greater attention in the development of intervention strategies to improve health outcomes and cultural recovery of best practices in wellness and preventative medicine. MLGBTQ2S American Indians experience many transitions in their lives, from rural and reservation living with grandparents, to having divorced or single parents, to urban detachment from Indian family and relatives. As one study respondent reported,

> Well my parents were divorced when I was three, so I was raised by my grandparents in Watsonville. So it was like . . . They were tired after raising fourteen children and several of their brothers' and sisters' kids. They were just like, "We love you, go play." So it was like, "Stay away from that freeway!" "Stay away from some other people too." But . . . yeah, just doing the chores, going to school, get good grades, go to sleep. So, like, it was hard. It was like they were tired—they didn't give us all the time and attention that we need, so they were not a very demonstrative family. I guess Navajos are kinda that way, pointing with your chin. So it was like a lot of hugging and stuff but more attention about the problems was needed when I was growing up. There was also a lot of food, good food too.

Another participant's story included some similar elements:

> I was raised in San Francisco, for the most part. Four years in San Diego, and um . . . my parents divorced when I was young. I was raised mostly by my mom's side of the family, which is not the Indian side. That was the Portuguese and Asian side. And um, I had some contact with my dad but it was

sort of minimal, here and there. . . . Basically when I went to college that
was when I started investigating more of my Indian culture and that's when I
went back to Oklahoma, got enrolled, and met more of my family, and started
interacting more with them. During this time I also started working my first
job here at the Native American AIDS Project, after college. And that job, in
addition to me attending an Indian community college was my next sort of
introduction into the Indian community. But my first step was family in Oklahoma during college, and then the Indian community college, and then here
at NAAP."

The quotes above reveal subtle and yet important aspects of radical love
as a central healing theme for Native peoples facing the ongoing impact of
colonial haunting and intergenerational trauma. One participant found that
love was demonstrated through hugs and perhaps not always by words or
direct communication, as is not uncommon in some Native families and tribal
contexts. The other participant found himself after being disconnected from
his Native identity by attending a tribal college, meeting his family in Oklahoma, and working with an ethnic-specific HIV/AIDS health organization,
a process that reveals the need for greater networks of support, community
cohesion, and cultural recovery within urban MLGBTQ2S communities in the
San Francisco Bay Area.

There is currently an expanding body of research literature within the field
of health geography that focuses on the therapeutic benefits of land and place
in the wellness of Indigenous peoples in the Americas. But research among First
Nations groups in Canada, for example, reveals a continuing lack of substantive
research on therapeutic landscapes as more than physical or symbolic locations of healing (Wilson 2003). First Nations peoples argue that relationships
with the land shape the cultural, spiritual, emotional, physical, and social lives
of individuals and communities. Similarly, geographic research has explored
First Nations peoples' health, but few studies have attempted to examine the
influence of cultural beliefs and values on health—not to mention the complex
linkages between the land and health (Wilson 2003). Connecting land to values
and health ultimately requires a concentrated effort to restore culturally specific
beliefs and practices into daily life, until there is no distinction between the
physical, emotional, and spiritual wellness of all living beings. This restoration
process is another way that I define radical love, as the activation of a deeply
embedded and reciprocal devotion to holistic and ethnic-specific self and community care through a balance of human feelings, emotions, and practices that

reduce egocentrism while emphasizing the symbiotic relationship between the physical and spiritual realms as co-constitutive factors of health promotion among Indigenous peoples.

MLGBTQ2S American Indians can reduce the health risks associated with historical and intergenerational trauma by restoring practices of radical love as a way to align the physical and spiritual dimensions of human existence. This means—as I began this chapter—that vulnerability, as an aspect of radical love, can heal spirit-traumas and other ongoing effects of intergenerational trauma, if and when cultural recovery and ethnic-specific therapies are developed, defined, and led by Indigenous peoples themselves.

Restoration of Indigenous knowledge and cultural practices will go a long way in reducing health disparities within Native populations, especially among mixed-bloods, who often cite cognitive dissonance and ethnic pulls between the different aspects of their identities as barriers to their health (see chapter 5). Gender and racial discrimination must also factor into the restoration process, as MLGBTQ2S Natives report high levels of gender and racial discrimination at various points in their lives. Chapter 4 examines in greater detail the contours of gender and racial discrimination as key components of the psychosocial risk factors experienced within this unique ethnic demographic. The IBPN risk model shows how Two-Spirit cultural dissolution is exacerbated by additional psychological and social factors such as historical and intergenerational trauma and gender and racial discrimination. Connecting cultural recovery and ethnic-specific leadership to land, health, and wellness will provide an important avenue for reducing stress and high-risk sexual behavior for MLGBTQ2S people who seek out ethnic-specific organizations like NAAP to provide them with an urban Indian kinship network of support.

CHAPTER 4

Gender and Racial Discrimination against Mixed-Race American Indian Two-Spirits

I didn't have a good relationship, I guess, with all the
men in the family. I'm the one that likes to lead and sing and
dance in the backyard and talk to the animals. . . . The men in
my family were all like, "sissy." . . . I didn't know that I was gay,
I just knew that I was different. I mean, who else runs around
singing Snow White songs? Little boys running around singing
Snow White songs, feeding the chickens . . . that was me!

—Indian Blood focus group respondent

DISIDENTIFICATION AND THE POLITICS
OF NATIVE IDENTITY(IES)

The socially constructed nature of gender and race in the United States has had
an enormous impact on the ways that LGBTQ people come to understand and
define themselves as masculine, feminine, butch, femme, or genderqueer, and
as male, female, transgender, Two-Spirit, et cetera. The rigid nature of these
gender and race categories causes many forms of isolation and social alien-
ation that place MLGBTQ2S people in awkward, threatening, and uncomfort-
able situations, as illustrated in the quotation above from one of the research
participants. To perform gender, as Butler (1993) suggests, is to understand
that our gender is a product of what we do at particular moments in time, and
that it is as much culturally based as it is biological and socially constructed.
There is no universal way to do gender: "There is no gender identity behind
the expressions of gender . . . identity is performatively constituted by the very
'expressions' that are said to be its results" (Butler 1993: 25). In other words,
what we do is what defines gender, not the other way around. Gender does not

dictate what nor how we do what we do as individuals. According to Butler, "one is not born a woman, but rather becomes one" (25). This position recognizes the fluid nature of gender and the agency that evolves from participating in a range of gender categories. MLGBTQ2S American Indians define their own experiences with gender and race in ways that often align with what Muñoz (1999) terms disidentifications.[1] Disidentification, unlike identification and counteridentification, is a strategic attempt to rework individual subjectivity in ways that challenge the socially constructed nature of identity categories. Muñoz explains that "to disidentify is to read oneself and one's own life narrative in a moment, object, or subject that is not culturally coded to "connect" with the disidentifying subject. It is not to pick and choose what one takes out of identification. It is not to willfully evacuate the politically dubious or shameful components within an identificatory locus. Rather, it is the reworking of those energies that do not elide the "harmful" or contradictory components of any identity. It is an acceptance of the necessary interjection that has occurred in such situations" (12).

Thus, to disidentify is to rework the meaning of one's identity for one's self and one's community in ways that are congruent with lived experiences, cultural practices, and the particular sociopolitical events that shape the trajectory of life stories for queer people of color. Many of the participants in the Indian Blood project speak to this notion of disidentification as a strategic attempt to reconcile the various identities that they hold as mixed-blood, LGBTQ, and/or Two-Spirit-identified Natives. Challenges to disidentification within this population are quite unique, given the extra-legal ways in which Native identity and group membership are defined through enrollment and sovereign, federally recognized tribal status. Rejection of tribal membership or disidentification with sovereignty for example can and often is read as a rejection of Native self-determination. Furthermore, identification as Two-Spirit can potentially be read as a disidentification with normative definitions of Native gender categories, as a result of gender stigmas enforced by colonial policies and practices. In other words, to disidentify or rework one's identity in new forms can challenge the legitimacy of already fragile ethnic, legal, and gender diverse formulations within American Indian communities.

Adapting to power, as Muñoz's work suggests, is a negotiation of strategies of resistance, as discourse and power fluctuate and shift over time and during particular political moments. Non-Native people, however, hold a privilege when it comes to disidentification that is not available to most Native people. In the United States, where American Indians are the smallest of the major racial groups and also the least visibly represented within the political arena, any form of disidentification becomes read as anti-Indian, or as a threat to the legal and sovereign status of Indigenous peoples in this country. For example, identifying as mixed-blood has been sharply criticized by Native scholars such as Elizabeth Cook-Lynn (1996). Cook-Lynn states that self-described mixed-blood writers such as Gerald Vizenor, Louis Owens, Wendy Rose, Maurice Kenny, Michael Dorris, Diane Glancey, and others produce writings that give much lip service to the condemnation of America's treatment of the First Nations, but she also asserts that "there are few useful expressions of resistance and opposition to the colonial history at the core of Indian/White relations. Instead, there is explicit and implicit accommodation to the colonialism of the "West" that has resulted in what may be observed as three intellectual characteristics in fiction, non-fiction, and poetry: an aesthetic that is pathetic or cynical, a tacit notion of the failure of tribal government as Native institutions and of sovereignty as a concept, and an Indian identity which focused on individualism rather than First Nation ideology" (58).

These oppositions—individual versus collective and mixed-blood versus traditionalist—are somewhat dated. Yet they continue to go unresolved in many ways because there is a lack of critical theorization regarding the ability of mixed-blood Natives to use approaches like disidentification to strengthen tribal sovereignty—not as a mirror image of Western heteropatriarchy, but rather as a set of kinship and citizenship systems based on the assets of each individual, regardless of degree of Indian blood, making the collective stronger. It is important to find the balance between situating mixed-blood/mixed-race Native identity and gender diversity within tribally specific contexts and the essentialist position that could be attributed to Cook-Lynn's assertion. Cook-Lynn's argument can reinscribe a form of nationalism that reduces Native identities to one form, as if there were one universal Native nation sharing one collective memory and one experience with colonization. But not all American Indian nations were removed, not all tribes were conquered through war, nor have all tribes lost their languages. Diversity always existed within the Native nations of the Americas, from the organization of tribes (patrilineal or matrilineal), to distinct clan systems, to gender categories (numbering from two to four or more), to use of the land, to ceremonies, to foodways, to phenotypes. This traditional diversity still exists, albeit eclipsed by extra-legal narratives that constrain both identification and counteridentification.

MLGBTQ2S American Indians resist the notion of a singular or uniform gendered and racialized set of Native identities. As Muñoz explains, "disidentification negotiates strategies of resistance within the flux of discourse and power" (19). MLGBTQ2S Natives employ ongoing strategies of resistance against the social arrangements that keep them confined to the margins of both mainstream U.S. and tribal politics. These experiences of marginalization and racial and gender ascription produce the conditions for racial and gender discrimination against MLGBTQ2S people. Those who wish to understand issues of agency and responses to power among marginalized populations must, as Muñoz argues, "understand that counterdiscourses, like discourse, can always fluctuate for different ideological ends and a politicized agent must have the ability to adapt and shift as quickly as power does within discourse" (19). The Indian Blood research data indicates that participants as a group experience extremely high levels of both racial and gender discrimination as a result of colonial haunting, racism, sexism, economic inequalities, transphobia, and homophobia. Disidentification has limits as a strategy for reducing or transforming these multiple forms of discrimination because it requires a deeper understanding of Native American identity among the general population and an acceptance among mixed-race Natives that they can self-identify as both Native and another race, without the other identity always superseding the Native identity in medical importance, visibility, and social acceptance.

Scholarship in the field of public health supports the argument that discrimination impacts the physical and mental health of American Indians and puts them at greater risk for long-term health disparities, including HIV/AIDS, through microaggressions, daily acts of injustice conveyed by both verbal and nonverbal messages suggesting that Native people and people of color are inferior groups (Walters, Evans-Campbell, Simoni, Ronquillo, and Bhuyan 2006). These often subtle acts of discrimination are categorized by Sue and his coauthors as microinsults (body gestures that suggest disagreement with or disdain for American Indian people who seek health services), microinvalidations (miscategorizing or dismissing American Indians as a vulnerable, at-risk population in need of medical services), and microassaults (direct statements or comments that undermine or make fun of American Indians and the health, gender, and race-specific issues they face) (Sue, Capodilupo, Torino, Bucceri, Holder, Holder, Nadal, Esquilin 2007). Gender and racial discrimination can be mitigated through stress-coping mechanisms that range from substance abuse to exercise to participation in cultural activities. Not every form of stress-coping equally reduces high-risk sexual behavior. In fact, as we will see below, some stress-coping strategies actually can increase risk for HIV/AIDS transmission among members of this demographic.

GENDER DISCRIMINATION AND STRESS-COPING
AMONG MLGBTQ2S NATIVES

A 2012 report, "Injustice at Every Turn: A Look at American Indian and Alaskan Native Respondents in the National Transgender Discrimination Survey,"
reveals that American Indian and Alaskan Native transgender and gender nonconforming people face extremely high levels of discrimination when compared with all other transgender and gender nonconforming people by race
and ethnicity (National Gay and Lesbian Task Force 2012). Among the report's
key findings:

- American Indian and Alaskan Native transgender and gender nonconforming people often live in extreme poverty, with 23 percent reporting a household income of less than ten thousand dollars per year, as compared to15
  percent for transgender people of all races. This rate is about three times
  that of the general American Indian and Alaskan Native population rate (8
  percent), and nearly six times the general U.S. population rate (4 percent).

- American Indian and Alaskan Native transgender and gender nonconforming people had a very high unemployment rate, at 18 percent, well over twice
  the rate of the general population (7 percent) at the time the survey was
  fielded.

- American Indian and Alaskan Native respondents who attended school
  expressing a transgender identity or gender nonconformity reported alarming rates of harassment (86 percent), physical assault (51 percent), and
  sexual assault (21 percent) in grades K–12; harassment was so severe that it
  led 19 percent to leave school.

- American Indian and Alaskan Native transgender and gender nonconforming
  people were affected by HIV in devastating numbers: 3.24 percent reported
  being HIV positive (an additional 8.53 percent reported that they did not
  know their status). This compares to rates of 2.64 percent for transgender
  respondents of all races, and 0.60 percent for the general U.S. population.
  Fifty-six percent of American Indian and Alaskan Native transgender respondents reported having attempted suicide, compared to 41 percent of all study
  respondents. (Quintana, Fitzgerald, Grant 2012: 1–2)

Data findings from this national study are consistent with the levels of discrimination found among the MLGBTQ2S participants I spoke with throughout the
course of my research with NAAP. Among the fifty Indian Blood participants,

36 percent stated that they had experienced gender discrimination at varying rates during a six-month period, while a slightly higher number, 40 percent stated that they had experienced gender discrimination on a daily basis during a twelve-month period.

Of the 36 percent of participants who reported gender discrimination during a six-month period, the average number of experiences with some form of gender discrimination was ten encounters (i.e., nearly twice a month). For some participants, encounters with gender discrimination occurred on a daily basis and deeply impacted their self-esteem, as well as their social and community engagement with peers and family members. Many of the male participants, for example, described being more comfortable with queer females than with other men, as a result of gender discrimination that takes a unique form against gay, queer, bisexual, and transgender men. One participant's comments about his physical appearance and comfort around "dykes" speak to the power of gender discrimination and historical trauma related to sexual violence to isolate MLGBTQ2S Natives from having healthy sexual relationships:

> I'm short, I'm fat, and I'm red. And I ain't upset about it. When it comes to dominant culture I've never related. I mean never. I always look at values— well on the contrary, I kind of take an opposing view, is that what they call it? Identity to me is still kind of problematic because of quote "gay/queer" culture. I was never "out," but I was labeled as being out, so I was the person that other people came out to, both male and female. Historically, I've always, ALWAYS, been at more comfort with um . . . female identity. Whether it's biological, mostly biological female, but it's just that femaleness. If I've got a choice, if I'm gonna kick it with the boys, hetero or gay or queer, or I'm gonna kick it with the dykes, I'm going with the dykes. 'Cause I can relate, I understand those dynamics.

Never relating to dominant culture can be both empowering and isolating. But always living your life as an outsider because your gender, race, and sexuality mark you as inferior is an ongoing problem inherited from the colonial period that continues to contribute to intergenerational trauma, violence, and silence about the ways that power in gender and sexual relations is used to oppress, damage, and alter the self-perception of MLGBTQ2S Natives. The same participant who expressed more comfort around "dykes" and a discomfort around other gay or queer men had a history of sexual violence from a very young age:

At the age of eight, I started, or I was being raped. I was raped from the age
of eight until I was eighteen. Right or wrong I actually did the one thing that
they tell you not to do and I actually resisted, so I experienced some extreme
violence. I suppose I'm kind of a case study. I was just eight when this all
started. So the behavior that I took on, displayed, during that time, was
atypical. I tried to resist. But yet it's in the American paradigm, let's blame
the victim, and I was just a bad student. And it's like, no, I was just doing the
best I could with, you know, I was just doing the best that I knew how given
the circumstances. Later I got into the BDSM [bondage, dominance, sado-
masochism] world. Hmmm, I wonder why? BDSM. Pain baby, pain! But you
know, I was more comfortable with the androgynous aspect of it. . . . But then
. . . that's when gender-fucking really kind of started to emerge and that's
where—whether they were biological male or female, we were gender fuck-
ers. So I've never identified really with "gay," maybe because growing up I was
painted as being gay. And being "gay" meant being "weak" or a "sissy"—like
a girl. That's not anything like the women I know. So when people ask me if
I'm "gay" it's like, do I look fucking happy to you? You know? And I don't [look
happy].

Other people, mostly men, projected a female gender onto this mixed-race,
Two-Spirit identified man because, as Andrea Smith suggests in her 2005 book
Conquest, "violence against Native women is inextricably linked to the state.
Indian bodies have become marked as inherently 'dirty' through the colonial
process. They are then considered sexually violable and 'rapeable,' and by
extension, Native lands become marked as inherently invadeable. That is, in
patriarchal thinking, only a body that is 'pure' can be violated. The rape of
bodies that are considered inherently impure or dirty does not count" (31–52).

Gender discrimination against MLGBTQ2S people comes from a long history of state-controlled, legally embedded and institutionally constructed
gender projects that seek to emasculate queer men, oppress Native women
and women of color, and to hypersexualize all people of color and Indigenous
peoples regardless of sexual orientation. That more than one-third of the study
participants reported experiencing gender discrimination over the course of a
twelve-month period indicates an extremely high and potentially disproportionate rate of gender oppression for MLGBTQ2S people.

In addition to high levels of gender discrimination, survey data yielded
interesting results regarding changes in gender identification over time.
Twenty-eight percent of the MLGBTQ2S participants reported experiencing

some change over their lifetimes in how they self-identified in terms of gender. As a whole, 64 percent of participants had identified their gender as male, 22 percent as transgender, 8 percent as Two-Spirit, 4 percent as female, and 2 percent as intersex. While we might assume the majority of transgender participants had experienced some change in their gender identity over time, this still does not account for the remaining 6 percent of participants who reported having had a shift in their gender identification. Two-Spirit and intersexed individuals also experience nonheternormative gender identity development, so while it cannot be confirmed this may be where we can assume that the other 6 percent who experience a change in gender identity are coming from as a combination of identity groups (transgender, Two-Spirit, intersexed). This speaks to the shifting ways that MLGBTQ2S American Indians are decolonizing and reworking notions of gender identity beyond male, female, and transgender to include Two-Spirit, as an act of cultural revitalization on the one hand and of resistance on the other.

These patterns of gender discrimination among MLGBTQ2S Natives are consistent with other psychosocial elements included in the IBPN risk model. Like Two-Spirit cultural dissolution, historical/intergenerational trauma, and racial discrimination, gender discrimination exacerbates social stigma, isolation, and high-risk sexual behavior. Poor health outcomes have been shown to be directly related to discrimination and marginalization based on sexual orientation, gender, and race (Fisher and Fisher 1992; Diaz 1997; Fergusson, Horwood, Ridder, and Beautrais 2005). When we observe every indicator for quality of life, Indigenous peoples in the United States and around the world are regularly overrepresented in rates of mental illness, disease, and overall morbidity rates (Fergusson, Horwood, Ridder, and Beautrais 2005). In addition to the prejudicial treatment that MLGBTQ2s American Indians and other queer people face on the basis of their sexual orientation, colonial and settler-colonial narratives within the broader society signal to non-Natives that it is "fair and reasonable to discriminate against people because of their sexual orientation. The consequences of this inequitable treatment have a negative impact on the people at whom the discrimination is leveled, as well as on the broader communities from which these people come" (Aspin 2011: 119). Aspin's assertion is useful in understanding the power of gender and sexuality discrimination not only on individuals, but also on entire communities already marginalized on the basis of race and class. When any person of color's community also internalizes colonial narratives about sexuality and gender, the resulting discrimination materializes as internalized oppression. MLGBTQ2S people need stronger community support from heterosexual-identified Natives and from their broader tribal and urban Native communities in order to buffer against the multiple forms of discrimination that increase their risk for HIV/AIDS and mental illness. The strategies we employ to address mental illness and HIV/ AIDS must take account of the multiple layers of psychosocial risk, including gender and racial discrimination, faced by MLGBTQ2S Natives.

RACIAL DISCRIMINATION AND STRESS-COPING AMONG MLGBTQ2S NATIVES

MLGBTQ2S American Indians do not separate racial identity from gender and sexual identity. When participants were asked how they thought their lives would be different if they were not mixed-race or queer, their responses indicated some acceptance of the social status quo. One participant said, "You know that's kind of like playing the 'what-if' game. And I don't know . . . for me what I've experienced in life has made me who and what I am and the fabulous [person] that I am. So to not have those experiences as . . . harsh and tragic as they were . . . to me it's almost kind of disrespectful to even [consider it]. I never wanted to be anybody else, because that's not my path, that's not my role." This respondent had been through many violent and traumatic life experiences as a result of his mixed-race background and his sexuality, but his answer indicates an acceptance that all of it had a purpose in making him who he is today. While there is empowerment and agency in this statement, as well as a concrete example of the ways that being vulnerable and open can encourage healing in a mental health context by reducing the pain associated with spirit-traumas, there is also a sense of resignation in the participant's statement. He seems to be asking, "This is how it is, so what else can I do?"

In contrast, another respondent believed that his life would be different if he weren't gay, saying: "I think if I weren't gay, I also would not have HIV. I think I wouldn't have had unprotected anal sex and gotten HIV. I could have done it, but I think it would be very, very low percentage of people, straight people, straight guys, [some] do have HIV. . . . But the risks are completely different." This respondent conflates his HIV-positive status with being gay as a result of his acceptance of mainstream stereotypes that equate being gay with contracting HIV/AIDS. His answer shows how discrimination on the basis of gender and sexual orientation, coupled with racial discrimination, perpetuates self-fulfilling prophecies and racial and sexual pathologies regarding HIV/AIDS transmission.

For at least four decades, feminist scholars of color have argued that in order to fully understand the social, political, and cultural issues impacting Indigenous people and communities of color, we have to address questions of intersectionality, that is, how race and class also impact questions of gender discrimination. Several scholars link racial discrimination to health outcomes and health disparities among Indigenous people and people of color (Walters, Simoni, and Evans-Campbell 2002; Diaz and Ayalya 2011). When we turn to the colonial history of the United States, there is no greater racial dilemma when it comes to ethnic and racial "authenticity" than that found among American Indians. According to the Office of Federal Acknowledgement, charged with determining the legal federal status of American Indians under 25 CFR Part 83, Procedures for Establishing that an American Indian Group exists as an Indian Tribe, there are seven mandatory criteria must be met:

(a) The petitioner has been identified as an American Indian entity on a substantially continuous basis since 1900.

(b) A predominant portion of the petitioning group comprises a distinct community and has existed as a community from historical times until the present.

(c) The petitioner has maintained political influence or authority over its members as an autonomous entity from historical times until the present.

(d) A copy of the group's present governing document including its membership criteria. In the absence of a written document, the petitioner must provide a statement describing in full its membership criteria and current governing procedures.

(e) The petitioner's membership consists of individuals who descend from a historical Indian tribe or from historian Indian tribes which combined and functioned as a single autonomous political entity.

(f) The membership of the petitioning group is composed principally of persons who are not members of any acknowledged North American Indian tribe.

(g) Neither the petitioner nor its members are the subject of congressional legislation that has expressly terminated or forbidden the Federal relationship (Bureau of Indian Affairs 2013).

No other ethnic group in the United States is expected to meet such strict criteria in order to prove membership. These criteria produce challenges around membership, enrollment, and disenrollment for many Natives, especially those disqualified on the basis of racial or gender discrimination. As Joanne Barker (2011) argues, the "Indian tribe," is the most studied and scrutinized ethnic group in the United States as a result of the process of federal recognition, which, at least technically "indicates that Native groups possess federal status and all commensurate rights under the law, including the right to self-government, sovereign immunity, and tax exemption" (27). As Barker points out, though this process in theory works fine, in practice the federal recognition category actually confuses and blurs the lines of federal and tribal nation-state authority: "But, ideologically, it is a category that works in far more obscure ways to provide for the continued rearticulation of federal authority over Native peoples. It is, in other words, most certainly not about who is and is not recognized so much as it is about the ongoing processes of social formation that work to keep Native peoples subjugated to U.S. power." The U.S. apparatus of control can be traced through a genealogy of colonial practices and policies to racial discrimination against American Indians in the present moment.

Indian-white relations involve a complex process of incorporation wherein Natives have always had to act in response, and defensively, when defining who they are and in maintaining their culturally distinct practices and modes of self-governance and group membership (Cornell 1990). The enrollment process of the late nineteenth century began a process of systematically excluding and legally "erasing" American Indians with any degree of admixture. Scholars have termed this policy of "vanishing" Indians as a paper or bloodless form of genocide (Forbes 1993, Jolivette 2007). MLGBTQ2S Natives, as a result of this long history and their relationship with racial haunting and discrimination, encounter many obstacles to obtaining services and in maintaining ethnic identification with their American Indian communities. The disconnect between some urban American Indians and tribal reservation-based communities has led many to change the way that they identify their race at various points in their lives and for reason of self-preservation, for fear of being targeted as "impostor" or "wannabe" Indians. Even those with federal status, who hold enrollment cards and citizenship within federally recognized tribes, are challenged by the strict criteria to determine who is a "real Indian." Consistent with the lived experiences of other multiracial populations, many Natives, including those in this study, shift how they identify according to where they live, who they are interacting with, and how they are perceived by outsiders. Twenty-four percent of the Indian Blood research participants reported having experienced a change in how they identified racially or ethnically. The average age for this change was twenty-four, which is consistent with research on emerging adulthood and the identity development process, as a time when individuals can assert an adult identity separate from how their parents and/or family members have identified them throughout childhood and adolescence.

Racial discrimination, perhaps even more than gender discrimination, has had a profound impact on the MLGBTQ2S participants in this study: 52 percent of participants stated that they had experienced racial discrimination regularly during a six-month period, with several noting that they experienced racial discrimination on a daily basis. When asked if they had experienced racial discrimination during a twelve-month period, the number responding "yes" rose to 58 percent. Racial discrimination in and of itself does not cause macro-level disparities in health, education, or class. But racism and its byproduct, racially discriminatory policies, are ongoing factors in the inequalities facing Natives and people of color in the United States.

Not linking racial discrimination to racism itself is an increasingly problem- atic feature of race theorization in the twenty-first century. In particular, the election of President Barack Obama signaled to many in politics, academia, and mainstream society alike that the United States was becoming a "colorblind society" in which issues of class discrimination were more salient than racism itself (Jolivette 2012). The discussion of class as causally predominant over race in producing oppression gains much of its traction from the work of sociologist William Julius Wilson, particularly *The Declining Significance of Race: Blacks and Changing American Institutions* (1980).[2] The work of Wilson, a key political advisor to President Bill Clinton in the late 1990s, contributed to a period of neoliberalism and race-neutral, colorblind policies that continue to perpetuate myths about racial progress in U.S. society. More recent works challenge this argument and speak to the defining feature of both racism and racial discrimi- nation: power. Sociologist Eduardo Bonilla-Silva, author of *Racism without Racists: Color-Blind Racism and the Persistence of Inequality in America* (2009), is clear about the role of power in defining racism in American society. In an interview with *The Grio*, an online African American media site sponsored by NBC, Bonilla-Silva is adamant that the concept of reverse racism is "nonsensi- cal," saying "when whites talk about reverse discrimination, I feel that they are making a silly argument, because what they really want to say is that we, people of color, have the power to do to them what they have done to us from the thirteenth century." Bonilla-Silva acknowledges that some people of color are prejudiced against whites but points out that they lack the power to dis- criminate against whites on a massive scale: "We do not control the economy. We do not control politics—despite the election of Obama. We don't control much of this country."

Indian Blood study participants are deeply impacted not simply by racial discrimination, but also by racism itself. Racism in this case is rooted in a long history of what Scott Richard Lyons terms "rhetorical sovereignty" or the difference between a nation-people and a nation-state (Lyons 2000). Lyons asserts that an Indian view of sovereignty is concerned not just with individual rights or political procedures and policies, but with a whole way of life. Lyons cites the work of Deloria and Lytle to illuminate his point: "Self-government is not an Indian idea. It originates in the minds of non-Indians who have reduced the traditional ways to dust" (Deloria and Lytle 1984: 21). Lyons continues, "Self-governance is certainly the work of a state but not necessarily that of a people; a people requires something more. However, while self-governance alone may not constitute the whole part and parcel of sovereignty, it nonetheless remains a crucial component" (456). That American Indian sovereignty is not exacted neither entirely as a nation-people nor as a nation-state speaks to the ongoing problems of control, power, and racism embedded not just in law, but also in culture. In an Indigenous framework we interrupt and trouble nationalism by moving away from the nation-state, where government institutions and officials are placed at the center of sovereignty, toward the nation-people, where everyday people are at the center of sovereignty, decolonization, and a dismantling of both racial discrimination (micro-level) and racism (macro-level).

MLGBTQ2S American Indians offer a unique lens from which to consider sovereignty from an urban Indian, mixed-blood perspective. Gender and racial discrimination have impacted Indigenous peoples from the fifteenth century to the present, and sovereignty still has not reduced extreme disparities in the health and well-being of American Indian people. Decolonizing gender, sexuality, and mixed-race identity in the face of colonial haunting, HIV, and the limits of sovereignty means we must reimagine and rework the ways that we understand, define, and value citizenship, kinship, and land/home/nation—we must turn toward an ideology of nation-people. Given that the majority of American Indians do not live on reservations, within the boundaries of the tribal nation-state, that mixed-bloods make up a majority of the population (estimates put the number at 65–70 percent), and that LGBTQ and Two-Spirit Natives are increasing in number and visibility, how can we accept changing notions of race, gender, and sexuality and move toward a new sovereignty, one that expands the tribal nation-state and balances it with that of the nation-people?

TOWARD A NEW SOVEREIGNTY

The concept of sovereignty dominates discourse in Indigenous studies through-out the Americas and the Pacific. Sovereignty often works as both the greatest resource and the biggest impediment to community cohesion and self-deter-mination in Native contexts, because the framework for sovereignty in many Native communities and nations often mirrors U.S. standards of self-gover-nance (see Deloria 1970, Warrior 1995, Sturm 2002, and Barker 2005). In the United States there is a long history of exclusion and oppression against citizens and those denied citizenship in order to control the most valuable resources for the smallest, most powerful group. MLGBTQ2S people provide an important case study of how the most vulnerable members of an already marginalized population are further excluded by their own members in the hopes of achiev-ing greater social mobility, economic resources, and positive national visibility (see Cohen 1999).[3] Using MLGBTQ2S participants as a case study invites us to imagine a new form of sovereignty that I term inclusive ecological sovereignty (IES). IES brings together existing forms of self-governance and democracy, not only opening understanding about changes in the political economy under glo-balization, but also incorporating both the nation-people and the nation-state. Its goal is to produce an ecological process based upon mutual solidarity that places the most vulnerable group members at the center of tribal governance. In many ways IES is a synthesis of traditional Indigenous knowledge and cultural values with emerging changes in social conditions and community embodi-ments such as race, gender, and sexuality. Colliding systems of knowledge sit at the root of problems with achieving IES for those who exist outside the ethnic, gender, or racial norms of Indigenous nations and communities.

Reimagining gender and racial diversity in the urban, mixed-race, context of the twenty-first century requires changing the face of our communities in order to save our communities—in both a metaphoric and a literal sense. The U.S. government has always had a what Stephen Cornell dubs an "Indian problem" (1990). The first and original problem was securing Native land; once that was accomplished, a subsequent problem emerges and continues to this day: how to make the Indian disappear. Making Natives disappear has been a project of both racial and cultural disappearance. Changing cultural beliefs and values relating to gender, sexuality, religion, and membership all contribute to an internalized U.S. hegemonic form of sovereignty. A first step to achieving IES is to reestablish membership criteria based not on blood quantum and enrollment status but on kinship, cultural knowledge, and group participation. If one government continues to manipulate hundreds of other governments into replicating U.S. sovereignty as their own unique form of sovereignty, the resulting disappearances will eventually solve the remaining Indian problem. We will all vanish if we continue to exclude mixed-bloods; we will all vanish if we continue to measure membership based on blood quantum. We will further isolate and exclude cultural contributions by those who live and express their gender and sexuality in diverse, complex, and socially meaningful ways. These exclusions will also lead to our final disappearance.

Sovereignty, as Amanda Cobb (2005) notes, is referred to by Native scholars in nearly everything that we write, no matter the discipline, because the term continues to be so central in making meaning of Indigenous life today. I conclude this chapter on discrimination by looking at sovereignty in order to argue that gender and racial discrimination against MLGBTQ2S Natives are the result of internalized mainstream U.S. views of race and gender—and because the adoption and application of those views in relationship to tribal sovereignty has been damaging. A crucial element of sovereignty, as noted by Deloria (1970), is freedom, but as Osage scholar Robert Warrior suggests (1995), we must define what type of freedom we are talking about when it comes to sovereignty. Both the intellectual sovereignty proposed by Warrior (1995) and the cultural sovereignty proposed by Singer (2001) and Cobb (2005) are closely aligned with what I outline above as IES.

IES, like intellectual and cultural sovereignty, weaves traditional cultural practices and knowledge together with contemporary cultural and political issues that change over time. The primary point of departure between IES and other theories of sovereignty, however, is its specific focus on processes of inclusivity that make the most vulnerable citizens and community members central while also reimagining how we define citizenship and equality. I attempt here not just to offer a theory of tribal sovereignty, but also to point to steps that could reduce the number of Native people facing gender and racial discrimination—in addition to numerous other stigmas—as a result of government policies and social processes that continue to exclude racial minorities, queer people, women, and people living with mental and physical health disparities. IES may also be the most practical solution for dealing with mixed-race cognitive dissonance among mixed-race American Indians, who make up the largest percentage of the American Indian population. Without a challenge to the federal government's authority to force tribes to maintain a membership system based on blood quantum and enrollment, there will be continue to be negative outcomes both for MLGBTQ2S people, who face multiple forms of marginalization, as well as for Indian nations themselves, which may face a crisis in membership if standards do not become more inclusive.

CHAPTER 5

Mixed-Race Identity, Cognitive Dissonance, and Public Health

Racially, I'm like a quarter white, but I don't feel white
and I don't look white, so people can't tell. . . . My dad, on the
Cherokee side, he was racist. He did not like Black people.
And I'm not sure if that was a part of being white or part of the
Indian side. And I sense . . . it's probably both. So I not only
experienced racism . . . but I also saw people in my own family
discriminating against other members of the family.

—Indian Blood focus group respondent

MIXED-RACE PEOPLE AND THE POLITICS OF MULTIRACIAL IDENTIFICATION

Identification as multiracial brings with it a multitude of potential challenges, even in 2016. While there is a growing body of literature on the subject of mixed-race identity and an even more promising body of work focusing on critical mixed-race studies, people of mixed descent continue to experience a high degree of cognitive dissonance and ambivalence as a result of the perceived power and privilege they are able to obtain by occupying multiracial spaces. One form this dissonance can take is what I term the mixed-race metronomic subject, an individual who is assumed to identify mechanically or unvaryingly with the same race just as a metronome is used by musicians to produce fixed beats. The mixed-race metronomic subject is socialized to perform a fixed, mechanical identity that never changes and that fits the expectations of both outsiders and insiders. MLGBTQ2S Natives often feel unidentifiable (as did the respondent above), and as a result many feel both conscious and unconscious pressure to surrender their power to name themselves in an ethnic/racial sense, because other people will always expect the mixed-race subject to respond to the same fixed identity that they ascribe upon them. The process of ascribing ethnic and racial identities upon MLGBTQ2S individuals also produces challenges in developing a congruent, collective social memory and sense of true community membership.

Here the properties of "Indian blood" become the metaphorical and literal mechanism through which power is able to speak. Foucault, in *Power/ Knowledge* (1972), states that "power speaks *through* blood; it is a reality with a symbolic function" (147). In this instance, I reframe Foucault's theorization in a contemporary Native American context, to suggest that "blood" is being used to define both race and social location based on race. If an individual assumes multiple bloods and therefore has stakes in multiple racial groups and social locations, it becomes very difficult, if not impossible, for "blood" to be used to signify membership. This is also complicated by the colonial process, which forcibly created a "new beginning" in the social memory of Indigenous peoples in the Americas. In Latin America, Canada, the Caribbean, and the United States, the history of racial mixing between American Indians, Africans, Europeans and Asians shifts the histories of Native peoples, forming a new social memory that throughout the course of more than five centuries becomes rooted in new formations and assumptions about the authenticity of memory, membership, and recollection of a primordial set of identities. Thus, when we recall an Indigenous past, we are also painfully recalling a colonial existence of often forced racial mixing, assimilation, removal, termination, and relocation. In his book, *How Societies Remember* (1989), Paul Connerton speaks to the "arbitrariness" of marking a new beginning because, as he suggests, the beginning has nothing to hold on to: "All beginnings contain an element of recollection. This is particularly so when a social group makes a concerted effort to begin with a wholly new start. There is a measure of complete arbitrariness in the very nature of any such attempted beginning. The beginning has nothing whatsoever to hold on to; it is as if it came out of nowhere. For a moment, the moment of beginning, it is as if the beginners had abolished the sequence of temporality itself and were thrown out of the continuity of the temporal order (6)".

In this instance the beginners are the mixed-bloods, who disturb and disrupt the continuity of the temporal order. There is no mixed-blood without colonization and its aftermath of colonial haunting. The generations of historical and intergenerational trauma then rest on the necks of the mixed-race subject, who is forever reconciling the past, present, and future. Belonging in the contemporary colonial moment suggests a specific ordering of group membership, based upon a set of fixed criteria that assume that certain bodies hold more cultural knowledge and investment in Indigenous self-determination. The irony of racial mixing is that many mixed-race subjects in fact challenge the metronomic, fixed pattern of self-identification and at the same time take on a form of social memory that is rooted in precolonial identity and preserving the cultural traditions of all sides, of all ancestries, so that they will not be challenged by other group members about their place within the community. For example, one participant's comments about language within his family demonstrate that assumptions based on degree of blood are often misplaced and erroneous:

> I came from mixed sides on both sides of my family, so my mom's side was like mixed Portuguese, Spanish, and Asian, and white. Like with the Portuguese side and the Spanish side they were like white, ethnically. And then my dad's side is Indian basically, and my dad's father who is mostly white. . . . He's like a quarter Cherokee. And it was like reversed. My dad's mom was like three quarters Cherokee. Um . . . My dad's father actually spoke more Cherokee than—my grandmother probably knew more Cherokee but she didn't really speak it publically. She just did it privately. But my dad did more . . . my grandfather did more business outside. But he wasn't enrolled, and she was the one who was enrolled. And um . . . and so um . . . When you trace my blood quantum it's from my grandmother's side. From my dad's mother's side.

It is important to note that in this participant's family, the grandparent with a lower blood quantum spoke the Cherokee language more than the grandparent with a higher degree of Cherokee blood. Many mixed-bloods work to prove their identities in ways that others do not have to, and this can cause feelings of rejection, isolation, and dissonance. Many MLGBTQ2S Natives are constantly expected to demonstrate their "Indianness" in ways that others are not because of differences in degrees of blood. Thus, the mixed-race, urban Indian subject throughout modern U.S. history plays a vital public role in bringing greater visibility to issues facing Native communities and tribal nations, not just in urban areas, but on reservations as well.[1]

In addition to facing issues around community acceptance of their mixed-racial backgrounds, MLGBTQ2S American Indians, like other multiracial people, are only recently receiving attention in public health research, especially in studies focusing on health disparities among vulnerable groups. Important trends within the multiracial population signal not only continuing growth but an increasing need for research into the health and well-being of people of mixed descent. While I would not assert that the socially constructed category of race itself is useful in measuring health risks and outcomes, I would argue that the racialization of particular groups and their experiences with racial discrimination, residential segregation, and poverty can serve as pathways to oppression (Tashiro 2005). Therefore research investigating multiracial people should not be based upon studies of genetics, so much as upon the diversity of experiences that shape and impact the health of mixed-race people, who are projected to make up nearly 21 percent of the U.S. population by 2050 (Waters 2000).

The participants in the Indian Blood study experience their identities in both positive and negative ways. Several participants grew up in environments in which cognitive dissonance around racial and ethnic identification led their families to deny or hide their Indian ancestry as a means of self-preservation and protection. One participant explained that "we were raised as Mexicans. My grandparents were forbidden to get married. I guess my grandmother's father said, 'You can't marry him.' So they ran away. They came to California and got married, and had fourteen children." The participant went on to elaborate how he had discovered that he was actually Navajo:

> So we were raised Mexican. [My grandpa] changed his name, so he wouldn't be bothered or whatever. And so we were Mexican, so most of our childhood we were Mexicans. And I was like, "I don't like that music, I don't like that, I like opera, I like ballet!" I was very strange. My grandmother would say, "I love you but you're a very strange child." . . . But right before my grandmother passed away, she goes, "There's something you need to know 'cause it will matter to you. You're not Mexican." And she goes, "You're Navajo. Your grandpa's Navajo. You're all Navajo." On my mother's side we're Navajo too. But I didn't really have any contact with Native culture till I met another Native at the gay Pride thing, I was walking around by myself and I saw him and he goes, "Come here!" That was my first push into the Native culture. But um . . . you know, growing up it was very difficult not feeling part of anything because I didn't identify with being Mexican. And it turned out I wasn't Mexican all along. I'm Navajo.

Growing up mixed-race and Native produces emotional and psychological challenges because U.S. society still does not do an adequate job of addressing racism. Social scientists, for their part, generally examine racism as a set of ideas about race rather than focusing on its actual impacts (Bonilla-Silva 1997).

While there have been thousands of studies on the subject of race and racism since the 1920s, it remains a relatively new area of study (see Banton 1970, and Miles 1989 and 1993). Studies of multiracial identity are an even more recent field of scientific inquiry (see Kitano 1984, Spickard 1991, Root 1992, and Daniel 2001). The earliest studies of race and people of mixed descent come out of the eugenics movement and offer only pejorative and white supremacist ideas about the diminishment that would occur if whites were to intermarry with Natives, Blacks, Latinos, or Asians (for early and influential writing on eugenics and race mixing, see Knox 1850, de Count Gobineau 1853, Nott and Robins Gliddon 1854, Darwin 1871, and Stonequist 1937). Mixed-race American Indians have a long history of being miscategorized and erased from public records in order to understate the size of the American Indian population thereby draining Native communities of resources.[2] Native peoples themselves have been deeply impacted by the internalization of white colonial sentiments about race mixing, especially with Blacks (Blu 1980; Forbes 1993, Sturm 2002; Perdue 2003; Saunt 2005; Miles 2006; Sturm 2002; Klopotek 2011, 2012). As Brian Klopotek points out in his essay "Dangerous Decolonization: Indians and Blacks and the Legacy of Jim Crow," "One of the thorniest issues to negotiate with people I interview has been the place of Blackness in southern Indian communities. The subject quickly raises hackles because of the ways in which the presence of Blackness undermines claims to distinct Indian identity; as a result of this and other factors, anti-Black racism remains an unresolved internal and external conflict in the South" (179).

Indigenous studies and subaltern studies are engaging in increased dialogue about the meaning of *subaltern* and *Indigenous* as modalities that can potentially challenge historical and economic understandings of colonization, miscegenation, and global imperialism (Byrd 2011). As MLGBTQ2S Natives seek to assert their multiracial identities, they are embodying a subaltern framework, speaking back and against colonial narratives that seek to homogenize Native peoples while simultaneously erasing mixed-bloods from historical memory, not to mention the historical record. Acknowledging the internalization of these colonial narratives about racial purity, homogeneity, and anti-miscegenation becomes of paramount importance if we are to understand how colonial haunting becomes a daily experience for MLGBTQ2S American Indians, who are routinely policed and questioned not just about their sexuality and their gender but also about their racial authenticity. This anti-miscegenation framing adds to an already difficult set of factors that produce high risk for HIV among MLGBTQ2S Natives. When we recall the IBPN risk model, we observe the interconnected causal relationship between Two-Spirit cultural dissolution, historical/inter-generational trauma, racial and gender discrimination, mixed-race cognitive dissonance, sexual violence, and impaired stress-coping in urban Indian kinship networks. Each of these factors must be addressed with multi-directional, intersectional analysis of the ways that dominant/subordinate, imperialist/subaltern, settler-colonial/indigenous patterns of marginalization and oppression are reinscribed within already marginalized communities. These binary reinscriptions also negate the realities of heterogeneity in Indigenous communities and thus underestimate the impact of colonization on the relationships between Native peoples and other marginalized groups. Brian Klopotek (2012) argues for the importance of researching the tensions between homogenous and heterogeneous Indigenous community identity narratives within the context of Indian-Black relations:

> But the problem of antiblack racism in Indian communities presents a theoretical oversight in indigenous methodologies in a couple of ways. First, indigenous methodologies need to be able to account for indigenous peoples as entities with blurred boundaries and internal heterogeneity rather than as discretely bounded, homogeneous communities. While scholars have often acknowledged the blurred boundaries between indigenous and colonizing populations that result in *mestizaje*, middle grounds, and colonial domination in American Indian studies, we have only more recently become more careful about accounting for the ways in which Indian communities have come into contact with other marginalized groups and at times reproduced systems of oppression from the colonizers within our own communities. (179)

Unpacking these relationships between Indigenous, colonizing, and other marginalized populations is central to the project of decolonizing gender, sexuality, and mixed-race identity(ies) within Native communities and nations as well as among the rest of U.S. society. To attempt to self-identify as a mixed-race Native often disrupts the multiracial identity development process. MLGBTQ2S American Indians, like other multiracial people, seek some level of affirmation, acceptance, and fluidity as they process and articulate their identities in the face of societally induced dissonance and exclusion. Over the past thirty years, racial and ethnic identity development scholars and multiracial theorists have developed alternatives to the linear models first proposed for identity development among minority groups (Atkinson, Morten, and Sue 1979; Cross 1995; Helms 1995), shifting to social environment models that use a series of political, geographic, linguistic, cultural, and ecological factors to determine individual identification processes (Renn 2003, 2004; Root 1998; Wijeyesinghe 2001).

These emerging models build upon foundational works in mixed-race studies by Poston (1990) and Root (1990) that focus on the healthy and positive resolution of identity development for biracial and multiracial people; in the process, these scholars also counter previous research suggesting that cognitive dissonance or maladjustment would be permanent experiences for people of mixed ancestry. Of the two foundational models, Root's specifically addresses the issue of biracial and multiracial identity, suggesting that in the face of racism, mixed-race people can assert a new group identity. Root's model includes four potential resolutions to the so-called dilemma of mixed-race identification:

1.   Acceptance of the identity society assigns. Family and a strong alliance with and acceptance by a (usually minority) racial group provide support for identifying with the group into which others assume the biracial individual most belongs.

2.   Identification with both racial groups. Depending on societal support and personal ability to maintain this identity in the face of potential resistance from others, the biracial individual may be able to identify with both (or all) heritage groups.

3.   Identification with a single racial group. The individual chooses one group, independent of social pressure, to identify himself or herself in a particular way.

4.   Identification as a new racial group. The individual may move fluidly among racial groups but identifies most strongly with other biracial people, regardless of specific heritage backgrounds. (237–46)

Root's model offers important alternatives for mixed-race people seeking to disrupt a long history of challenges to self-identification as monoracial, biracial, or multiracial. MLGBTQ2S participants throughout the research process asserted their identification as Native, or as Native and mixed-race. Almost all of the participants would be classified as having chosen resolutions two, three, or four in Root's model. All of the participants, whatever process they chose, included their Native or tribal identity as a part of their self-identification. This is where the MLGBTQ2S American Indians diverge slightly from Root's model: even as they identify with a new racial group (biracial/multiracial), they maintain another identification that not only includes their Indigenous ancestry but makes it central. While some of the participants did struggle with gaps in cultural knowledge, either because they were raised by a non-Native parent or relative or because they were separated from their tribes, all took seriously the programs and services available to them in the Bay Area to strengthen their understanding of the diverse histories and cultures of American Indian people in the United States, through both tribally specific and "pan-Indian" lenses. I attribute this deep investment in identification as Native in part to the vast resources available in the San Francisco Bay Area, which produce a strong sense of Indigenous cohesion, cultural engagement, and urban kinship. As MLGBTQ2S American Indians search for community in the face of cognitive dissonance, these urban Indian kinship networks provide a set of cultural and social resources that enhance the very stress-coping mechanisms that can reduce or eliminate the high-risk behaviors that lead to HIV infection.

MLGBTQ2S NATIVES AND THE SEARCH FOR COMMUNITY

Respondents reported being able to find the resources they needed in San Francisco because ethnic-specific agencies like NAAP and BAAITS provide a set of services that nurture the development of a supportive community for MLGBTQ2S Natives. Organizations like these are extremely important, because finding community and kinship networks in an urban environment can mean the difference between living life on the streets, addicted to drugs, or having the opportunity for social and cultural growth among other Native people, who, despite coming from diverse tribal backgrounds, can still offer a space for positive identity formation among MLGBTQ2S individuals. Many of the participants I spoke with discussed the hardships they faced while growing up. The common thread, whether participants had been on the reservation, in another rural setting, or in cities, was traumatic and isolating experiences during their formative years. Those who did not grow up around a lot of other Native people, faced additional challenges because they were teased and victimized in school and they did not always have the necessary tools in their communities to deal with the ways in which they were being marginalized. As one respondent described,

> I didn't have many Native friends, but they were mostly, it was almost like a white, white neighborhood, and they use to pick on me, kick me and everything. They [other kids] would wait for me. They'd call me names, some called me a woman, and I was just afraid of school. Then I finally met another Indian guy, he was from San Francisco, he later moved to Fresno. Then when I went to college I thought it would be better, but it wasn't. It just continued. . . .

To manage all of this, I'd hide. I'd hide and go around a park or just to get
away. . . . I didn't wanna be picked on, so I ditched P.E. groups, I didn't wanna
shower in front of the boys. So I would pretend I was ill and tried to go to the
nurse's office. That's it.

This response demonstrates the ways that racial and gender discrimination along with mixed-race cognitive dissonance can leave many MLGBTQ2S
Natives without the community support system that they need to stay away
from high-risk behaviors such as drugs and alcohol. Other participants express
how problems at home made life difficult—so difficult that the first place that
young people may turn to ease their pain is drugs.

Well, for me there was domestic violence in the home. When I was young
my mom and dad used to fight a lot. My dad was an alcoholic, and um . . . so
growing up wasn't, you know, like the best thing for me. Because then by the
time I was a teenager I got hooked on drugs and alcohol, so you know, there
were these [drugs] readily available, you know, in my environment, so, um,
that's kind of how I dealt with my problems growing up, you know, living
where I was living, until I came here.

The colonial impact of historical and intergenerational trauma made it very
difficult for many participants to relate stories and events from their child-
hoods that did not include some form of violence, abandonment, loneliness, or
social isolation as the result of the actions of outsiders or members of their own
families or communities. One participant spoke quite candidly about having
grown up in a stable foster family in a community with lots of resources and
still feeling out of place in terms of her mixed-race identity: "My natural parents
abandoned me when I was two years old. . . . So I was raised in a foster home,
and, uh, we were spoiled kids. I'm the oldest out of two brothers and two sisters
and they spoiled us to the max. I mean we lived in a great big house, and it was
a very nice neighborhood, a lot of rich kids, and I had a great time. This was in
Anchorage. But people, I guess thought and most still think that I'm Caucasian,
not Native American at all, so it's . . . it's been difficult."

This participant's experience speaks to the importance of identifying the
specific resources that are most needed for positive identity development and
growth among MLGBTQ2S Natives. First, these resources should include access
to culturally competent counseling, preferably provided by an American Indian
health agency and facilitated by a Native counselor. Second, tribally specific

educational and cultural programs should be available, to increase self-esteem and self-awareness related to specific tribal and ancestral roots. Third, MLG-BTQ2S Natives need to be supported and encouraged to participate in Native or tribal-specific community activities and events. Participating in community events with other MLGBTQ2S American Indians provides a sense of belonging, something many participants reported having lacked during their adolescence. And fourth, MLGBTQ2S Natives must be able to obtain affordable and preventative health care at ethnic-specific organizations that can ensure that they do not fall through the cracks.

Ethnic-specific health agencies often take a holistic approach that is not limited to the patient-doctor relationship; they offer a community-inclusive model in which spirituality, culture, health, and education come together and many people in addition to the primary care doctor or counselor work to support the health and well-being of the client. One respondent spoke to the ways that Native American-specific health facilities are meeting her needs in terms of primary care and substance abuse: "Well, I have had no problems getting services. I go to the Native American Health Center, you know, for my medical care—if I need anything, I go there. If I need anything [else], I come here [to NAAP], you know, that's pretty much . . . you know the agencies that they have, there's even a treatment center for Native American people, you know, in San Francisco. . . . They have substance abuse programs, so they have an outlet also. So, you know, there's a community here, you know? It's good."

Because this participant is surrounded by other Natives, she feels added comfort in expressing any medical issues she may have. Perhaps more importantly, in this environment, individuals can find it easier to describe experiences with intergenerational trauma, which in another setting might go unaddressed because of Native distrust of non-Natives. The distrust of non-Native hospitals, researchers, doctors, and counselors is very much based in history and is deeply entrenched as a part of the ongoing process of colonial haunting that is often perpetuated by these very non-Native individuals and institutions. For example, physical abuse and the denial of food and/or medicine have been observed in studies of older Native Americans living in urban areas (Buchwald, Tomita, and Manson 2000). There is also a documented history of discrimination and negligent medical practices in research in Indigenous communities, including the forced sterilization of nearly 25 percent of American Indian women by 1977.[3] This long history of colonial abuse in health care and virtually every other sector of society has given many MLGBTQ2S Natives pause when it comes to seeking services at mainstream medical facilities.

While the majority of the Indian Blood participants did have access to ethnic-specific health services, either at NAAP or at the Native American Health
Center (NAHC) offices in San Francisco and Oakland, for other urban Indians access to adequate health care services continues to be a serious problem,
because individuals must be enrolled with a federally recognized tribe in order
to access care through Indian Health Service (IHS) offices. Further, most of
the nation's IHS facilities are located in remote rural areas or on reservations,
hundreds if not thousands of miles away from the cities where 67 percent of
Native people currently live, leaving them to fall through the cracks. Both these
factors—enrollment requirements among a population with high rates of interracial marriage and shrinking blood quantum percentages among younger
generations, along with the cost, distance, and time it takes to travel to HIS
centers—cause many to look to mainstream medical facilities or to ignore their
health problems altogether until serious issues present themselves (see Urban
Indian Health Commission 2007). In areas like San Francisco and Oakland,
eligibility requirements are less significant because organizations like NAAP
and NAHC allow anyone to use their services; they are not required by IHS to
use enrollment in a federally recognized tribe as a criteria for accessing services. Whether a given IHS facility requires proof of membership in a federally
recognized tribe is typically based on the percentage of IHS funding the agency
is receiving. During my time as a graduate student, the director of the NAHC in
Oakland shared with me that his center received the majority of their funding
from other sources than IHS, and therefore was not bound to the same enrollment criteria as most centers across the country. Between 2007 and 2008, under
the Bush administration, there was an attempt to completely eliminate all IHS
funding. If the Bush administration had been successful, this would have closed
more than thirty IHS centers across the country, leaving nearly 70 percent of
the 4.1 million American Indians and Alaska Natives without sufficient health
care. Public protest forced the administration to back down and the attempt to
cut the funding was eventually abandoned.

Today, the challenge for MLGBTQ2S Natives remains one of finding consistent community support to address issues of Two-Spirit cultural dissolution,
historical and intergenerational trauma, and racial and gender discrimination, among other struggles. Perhaps most importantly for promoting cultural
engagement as a stress-coping mechanism, they need ways to deconstruct
the centuries of mixed-race cognitive dissonance that have so often divided
nations, tribes, and communities. Some participants approach the subject of
mixed-race cognitive dissonance and community by following the third pattern

of identity development in Maria Root's 1990 model of biracial and multiracial identity development. In this pattern, as noted earlier, an individual "identifies with a single racial group. The individual chooses one group, independent of social pressure, to identify himself or herself in a particular way." Identification following this pattern can be described as a monoracial identification; however, the multiraciality of the individual may still be significant in how they are racialized by others. As one respondent described,

> As for me, um, I identify as Native American. I take part in the community. I go to, uh, social functions and events and things, um . . . that's my circle, and that's what I feel I am a part of. Um, sometimes, you know, like, a lot of Latino people think I'm Mexican or whatever and they speak Spanish to me or whatever . . . thinking that I'm Mexican. Um, my dad was Mexican and my mom is Native American, but I was not raised by my father's family, so . . . you know, I identify more as being Native American than anything else, because, you know, it's my circle.

Here, *circle* becomes a metaphor for a holistic, inclusive community. Consider that the participant says he participates in social functions and events. In these instances, he is receiving affirmation of his Native identity not simply as a result of his mother's lineage but because of his willingness and ability to participate in the community, his desire to be a part of the circle.

For other MLGBTQ2S participants, becoming a part of the circle meant learning about their Native identities and the Native community in general from friends who share similar social identity characteristics. One gentlemen in the study described his initial entry into Native communities as emerging from his friendship with a Native transgender woman.

> I did like I just said [move around to] different areas. I lived in Phoenix, and I ended up having some Indian trans friends. They're full Indian, I forgot what tribe they're from, but . . . And, like, that was my first experience where really, like, in my life . . . Honestly, having friends that are completely, totally Native American, you know what I mean? And they were such good friends. One friend of mine, her name was, uh, Sugar. . . . Yellow Hair, I think. She lived on the reservation and all. And so I got to learn a lot, like a lot, about it, and stuff. I never got a chance to go myself [to the reservation], 'cause it was like hundreds of miles away or something. . . . Yeah, so what I was telling you guys is that, um, that was, that was my first time, like even coming into contact with

the, um, Native American community, like as, you know, with friends. Like, you know, maybe professional [I have been in contact with before], but that doesn't really count, but like as, in personal, you know. . . . And I was accepted though—you know, they didn't turn me away just for [*sic*] I was mixed with something else.

The friendship this MLGBTQ2S man cultivated with another Native person who was transgender likely based on a certain level of empathy, as one identified as a mixed-race, gay American Indian and the other as a transgender American Indian. Having similar social identities creates the possibility for strong bonds to be forged, and for allies to be made. This man and his friend, Sugar, may both have experienced discrimination from others because of their Indian background, sexual orientation, and/or gender. Sharing experiences of discrimination and oppression can be a vehicle for bringing people together. MLGBTQ2S Natives who can form community relationships at the individual and group level are in a much better position to address stigmas associated with mixed-race cognitive dissonance. In fact, in the two previous examples, both mixed-race participants found ways to end any confusion they may once have felt about their place in and ability to participate in the American Indian community.

The overlapping of marginalized identities presents many participants with intense levels of stress and discrimination, as well as external pressures to live up to the racialized, gendered, and sexualized assumptions of non-Natives, particularly in institutional settings such as churches, hospitals, schools, and prisons. The pressure to live up to or dispel the assumptions of non-Natives is a daunting task, especially when it comes to living life as an HIV-positive person and/or as a transgender or mixed-race Native. One participant discussed the impact of religion as a stress factor in his life when it came to his gender, sexuality, and mixed-race background as Cherokee and African American:

So I am from West Virginia. Been out here for twenty-two years and I have Cherokee Indian on both sides of my family. Yeah, well from the religion that my family comes from it just wasn't acceptable, as far as my sexual preference. And you know, I've always been called a 'female.' And my mother always had to tell people that thought I was a female. I mean I didn't have to go through the process of taking hormones or anything like that. But it wasn't, um . . . difficult, really difficult for me until I came out here. And that's when some of the discrimination came about, you know. So I overcame that and moved on with my life, you know. I've been in and out of jail and prison, and that wasn't so easy. They sexually assaulted [me], before I came out here and while I was locked up. So it was kind of difficult sometimes you know. But I managed to push forward and talk about the things that affected me. And um . . . coming out was the biggest thing for me to find out who I was to myself . . . so it was so, so with me.

This individual and other participants face difficulties not just around coming to accept the various aspects of their identities, but also in facing and accepting their HIV-positive status and the stigmas that come from living with the disease. This process includes negotiating sexually intimate relationships and public perceptions about people who "look queer." One participant discussed how learning to cope with these stresses had led him to become a peer educator: "So ya know, being incarcerated . . . they have what they call 'jail house relationships.' I met someone else [in prison] that was mixed Indian. And I've been positive for twenty-two years. And, um . . . I'm still here by the grace of God. And I've always been an educator. People ask me, 'What are the symptoms or whatever?' And you know, I had that stigma, to where people were like, 'Eww! You're HIV positive?' So a lot of stuff like that, because you do get some people that act like that." While this person was able to use his HIV status to increase his involvement in the community, working to combat health disparities and stigmas around HIV-positive people, other MLGBTQ2S participants responded to their HIV-positive status with fear and silence to prevent rejection. This silence, however, often led to new problems, including incarceration:

I started dating when I was fifteen. Heterosexual women. I didn't get into transgenders, transsexuals, til I was eighteen. And it was a lot, way better. Well you know, I've been with one for ten years now. And as far as uh . . . like my family and friends they consider her 100 percent woman. And they're proud to know that she's Native American. And they just love her to death. There's never any problem with them, no nothing. And as far as sexual relationships, I always kept that pretty private and no one really asked about it. They respected my privacy. But there was one time . . . um, we had sex but I never wanted to cum inside of them [her] 'cause I don't know how she would react if I would've told her I was HIV-positive. Um . . . and we did this for about a month. Having sex, not cumming inside her. She tried to figure something out. . . . She would say, 'Like, you can cum inside me. I wanna have your baby.' And I said, 'I don't think you wanna have my baby.' Um, so um . . . So I was getting kind of worried and I think, you know, that since I was cumming on her, I thought, you know, that like the sperm would have went inside of her and she would have got HIV anyways. But . . . I um . . . So I had to leave to work and um . . . next thing you know, I came back. And she pressed charges on me 'cause I didn't tell her that I was HIV-positive. So I went to court and just felt bad about it. So, see my whole picture: I'm mixed, I'm brown, I'm HIV-positive . . . And um, yeah, I screwed up. First time ever I actually got charged, I think.

That this man did not have the courage to share his HIV-positive status with his sexual partner demonstrates how, despite medical advancements in treating HIV, stigma around the disease is still such that many choose to hide their status rather than face the potential loss or rejection of others. MLGBTQ2S individuals must also process the psychosocial factor of mixed-race cognitive dissonance, as we have seen throughout this chapter. It is clear that the overlapping factors of historical and intergenerational trauma, sexual violence, racial and gender discrimination, and Two-Spirit cultural dissolution can create greater high-risk behavior both for those who remain HIV negative and for those who are already living with the virus. MLGBTQ2S Natives who exhibit the greatest level of resiliency in the face of colonial haunting and the psychosocial factors of HIV risk are those who are the most comfortable in their ethnic/racial/gender identities and those who participate in the Native community and build solid relationships of support and urban kinship. Maintaining a sense of self-esteem in the face of so many different traumas and daily assaults on their psyches is no small feat for the MLGBTQ2S people who participated in this study. As chapter 6 highlights, sexual violence, like mixed-race cognitive dissonance, can weaken or destroy the coping mechanisms of MLGBTQ2S participants seeking to reduce their risk for HIV. But the following chapters also illuminate the powerful ways that religion, ceremony, and spirituality can be invoked to reconnect broken cultural and community ties, leading to healing for more and more people through the intentional formation of intergenerational healing and cultural leadership programs.

CHAPTER 6

Sexual Violence and Transformative Ancestor Spirits

I pray and I have an altar and I light that altar every
night . . . I just smoke 'em out with that sage and then I pray
about whatever I'm going through and I release it. I release it
into the universe. And then I open all the windows so it can just
blow out. . . . A lot of people should incorporate prayer with the
ancestors into their lives. We all need a higher power that we
can go to. To pray and release that negative energy
or whatever we're going through.

—Indian Blood focus group respondent

SEXUAL VIOLENCE AND HIV: AN "INVISIBLE" THREAT

MLGBTQ2S participants with a history of sexual violence were at the greatest risk for seroconversion to HIV. Among HIV-positive participants, 69 percent had also experienced some form of sexual violence. By comparison, the overall rate of sexual violence among all participants in the study was 56 percent. Examining sexual violence across gender and sexual orientation demonstrates the salience of sexual violence as an indicator of risk for contracting HIV. Among gay and queer-identified participants, 64 percent reported experiences with sexual violence, in comparison to 44 percent of bisexual participants, 77 percent of Two-Spirits, and 28 percent of transgender participants. One hundred percent of bisexual and Two-Spirit participants who were HIV positive had also experienced sexual violence. As suggested by the IBPN risk model, the psychosocial factors of Two-Spirit cultural dissolution, historical and intergenerational trauma, racial and gender discrimination, and mixed-race cognitive dissonance, when coupled with sexual violence, creates a system of multiple forms of marginalization that can be mitigated by stronger cultural buffers and stress-coping mechanisms. This chapter aims to examine how decision-making plays a role both in risk for HIV transmission and in patterns of behavior within Indigenous populations that continue to experience intergenerational trauma and sexual violence. I will later explore how affect theory can provide a framework for understanding risk behavior and HIV vulnerability among MLGBTQ2S populations.

Sexual violence against MLGBTQ2S populations has been overlooked in most research studies of violence within American Indian communities, as well in other communities of color. While there has been a significant amount of research within Native studies and public health on violence against American Indian women, there are very few studies that address sexual violence against gay, bisexual, and queer men. Equally problematic, government officials until very recently failed to address violence against American Indians and LGBT populations, despite staggering statistics that indicate disproportionate rates of violence against Native women, MLGBTQ2S Natives, and other marginalized groups. In fact, in 2012 the House of Representatives passed the Adams-Cantor (H.R. 4970) version of the Violence against Women Act (VAWA), which failed to include provisions to help immigrant, Native women, and LGBT communities. The vote was 222-205, with twenty-three Republicans voting against the bill and six Democrats voting for the bill. The 113th Congress took up VAWA again in January 2013. An inclusive VAWA that included provisions helping immigrant, Native American and LGBT victims of violence (S. 47) was passed in the Senate, and the House of Representatives approved it, 286-138. The bill was signed into law by President Obama on March 7, 2013.[1]

Because sexual violence against MLGBTQ2S individuals continues to be understudied, it remains a silent, "invisible" threat when it comes to receiving services for intimate partner violence and molestation, due to a lack of understanding from mainstream agencies about the specific needs of this community. Assumptions about violence that construct a narrative of only male perpetrators and female victims disregard the realities of intimate and domestic partner abuse that millions of LGBTQ people face every day. A study conducted by the National Coalition of Anti-Violence Programs in 2012 found that 45 percent of LGBT victims were turned away when they sought assistance from a domestic violence shelter. Nearly 55 percent of those who filed for protection orders were denied them.[2]

Domestic partner and intimate partner abuse, however, is only one aspect of the violence that MLGBTQ2S participants face. In fact, the majority of respondents spoke about sexual violence and molestation as children and young adults. One participant spoke about his first sexual experiences and the taboo surrounding incest: "And, um . . . my first experience with sexuality was with my deceased brother. And you know there was something forbidden. Like incest in the family. And so, I'm like, 'Okay bro, how do I cope with this?'" Incest and molestation continue to be sensitive subjects that many survivors of sexual violence are unable to speak about for years, if ever.

Sexual violence among MLGBTQ2S participants not only correlated with HIV positive status but also shaped the ways that respondents viewed dating and intimate partner relationships. One young man in the study spoke about sexual violence in his early years and how the race of his attackers plays a role in some of his current dating choices:

> I've got to say, I just thought of something. It's like, all the people that took advantage of me when I was young, that sexually abused me and raped me or whatever, it's like we're all . . . it's always, like, Mexicans. And the one that made me have sex with him at knife point was Native. He was Native, and he blackmailed me for four years, as I was Mormon, 'cause he was going to tell everybody. So I had to keep having sex with him, not wanting to—well, liking it, but not wanting to, you know? So it was like really weird, I just thought of that, and it's like, I guess that's like the White supremacist guy [who sexually assaulted me in the past].

This MLGBTQ2S individual's early experiences with sexual violence had an impact on how he viewed himself and potential dating partners on the basis of race and ethnicity. He felt less trust toward other Native men because of the violence he had experienced within his own community. Rebuilding trust in the face of sexual violence and colonial haunting proves difficult for many people who live through sexual violence, molestation, and/or incest.

The legacy of colonization as a process of state-sanctioned violence, including sexual violence, is revealed when we look more closely at rates of sexual violence by race and sexual orientation. According to a 1998 needs assessment, "Prevalence of HIV Infection in Transgendered Individuals in San Francisco" conducted by Clements, Marx, Guzman, Ikeda, and Katz (1998), 55 percent of female-to-male transgender people and 68 percent of male-to-female transgender people have been forced to have sex in their lifetime. Other research shows that while in the general population, 80–90 percent of incidents of rape against women are committed by someone of the same racial background, more than

80 percent of sexually violent crimes committed on reservations against Native American women are committed by non-Natives.[3] Gay men and lesbians are more likely to be raped than heterosexuals (about 12 percent for gay men and 31 percent for lesbian women report having been raped; in addition, they are more likely to be raped by strangers, often as part of physical assaults motivated by homophobia.[4] Research shows that sexual violence often leads to negative stress-coping mechanisms such as alcohol and drug abuse, which are in turn leading risk factors in the spread of HIV and AIDS (Browne and Finkelhor 1986).

Indian Blood participants exhibited high levels of engagement with both alcohol and drugs, and reported often having sex without protection. Their elevated rates of using alcohol and/or drugs during sexual encounters, like their elevated incidence rate of unprotected sex, may be explained by the high frequency with which members of the study group reported having experienced sexual abuse. Nearly 50 percent of all participants reported having engaged in unprotected sex during the past twelve-month period. Close to 60 percent had engaged in sex under the influence of drugs at some point in their lives, though rates of sexual activity under the influence of drugs or alcohol were slightly lower during the past twelve months.

According to Stall et al. (2003), men who have sex with men (MSM) living in urban areas experience increased risk for the co-occurrence of psychosocial health problems, which in turn put them at increased risk for HIV. These co-occurrent psychosocial health problems are known as syndemics and include factors such as partner violence (Greenwood, Relf, Huang, Pollack, Canchola, and Catania 2002), childhood sexual abuse (Paul, Catania, Pollack, and Stall 2001), and depression (Ciesla and Roberts 2001). Stall and his co-authors further argue that there is a relationship between these three psychosocial health problems and increased risk of HIV transmission.

> Finally, these data suggest that syndemic conditions are understudied phenomena in public health research. The lifelong effects of social marginalization or stigma may work to create high occurrence of psychosocial health problems among urban MSM, problems that in turn function in an additive manner to raise levels of high-risk sexual behavior and thus HIV infection itself. Thus, in some other populations, greater understanding of the mechanisms of disease interplay might also include study of the effects of malnutrition, stress, poverty, and racism, as well as homophobia. Research questions should address the basic public health question regarding syndemics: What are the best approaches to disrupting syndemics so that the health of vulnerable populations is enhanced? (942)

Syndemics, or co-occurrent psychosocial health problems that lead to the spread of disease, should be a primary concern for researchers in Indian Country. Public health scholars, particularly those studying HIV, must, as Stall concludes, examine the lifelong impact of social marginalization and stigma as each relates to the vulnerability of oppressed populations at risk for HIV and other diseases. As the empirical data reported above suggests, high rates of sexual violence, child abuse, and molestation among MLGBTQ2S Natives are correlated with elevated rates of risk-taking behavior that increase the probability for HIV transmission However, as the rest of this chapter explores, the Indian Blood study is not simply another tragic story of Native illness and suffering. Rather, it is also a collection of life narratives that offer important insights into how individuals of mixed-racial and ethnic ancestry who also identify as LGBTQ or Two-Spirit navigate and transcend the traumas of sexual violence as adults and in supportive intimate relationships.

TRANSCENDING THE TRAUMAS OF SEXUAL VIOLENCE

Many MLGBTQ2S participants indicate that transcending the traumas of sexual violence, emotional abuse, and intergenerational trauma involves cultivating positive relationships with other Natives, especially those who also come from mixed ethnic and cultural backgrounds. One participant described his own trajectory in these terms:

> I dated all sorts of guys and um . . . at twenty-one, I came out and, um, I didn't have really any sexual experience until about that time. And the first person that I had a sexual experience with is actually a high school friend. We were in the same class, and we met at a club and he said, "I want you to come home with me." And I said, "Okay." I sort of knew what was going on, but I wasn't sure [laughs] . . . and I think that was my first sexual experience. And it was here in the city, and um . . . I dated lots of different types of guys racially. The guys I felt I've loved and had the most deep relationships have been other mixed-race guys. Guys who are about a deeper understanding with, um . . . you can see both sides of being whatever, whatever racial makeup they were, they could see racial dynamics better. Usually it was the guys that were Indian and something else. And um . . . I feel more comfortable with people of color generally, even though I'm dating a white dude now.

The ability to transcend—or at least begin a process of healing from—trauma and sexual violence is dependent to some degree on emotional attachment. It

therefore involves anxiety around decision-making, as well risk-taking in relationships and intimate social, cultural, and/or sexual engagement.

Here, the work of affect theory scholars offers important insight into how
the individual and developmental processes of decision-making can contribute
to healing among adult survivors of sexual violence. According to Mellers and
her co-authors (1997), most studies of decision-making are silent about the
role of emotion in risk-taking. Mellers argues for what she calls "decision affect
theory," which examines decision-making from the perspective of the emotional attachment to expected outcomes when making decisions that involve
risk. She explains that "most theories of decision making treat choice behavior as a cognitive process; people assess their values, define their goals, and
take actions to achieve those goals. But anyone who ever made an important
decision knows that what really happens is not that simple. People often base
decisions on emotions. . . .We propose a theory of emotional experience that
we call decision affect theory. . . . It is a theory of postdecision affect rather
than choice" (Mellers, Schwartz, Ho, and Ritov 1997: 423). Knowledge of self
also plays a vital role in decision-making, particularly in the case of high-risk
decisions related to health outcomes, in which a history of sexual violence and
traumatic life events frequently comes into play. In other words, MLGBTQ2S
people who experience sexual violence and trauma are less likely to engage
in high-risk behaviors if they maintain a greater degree of self-awareness and
have addressed their past experiences through collective healing and wellness measures with an American Indian focus. The way that MLGBTQ2S participants described making these risky decisions demonstrates that they do
indeed weigh potential emotional setbacks, sometimes employing negative
stress-coping mechanisms such as drinking alcohol, taking drugs, or engaging
in unprotected sex.

Because the American Indian population is so small and is often overlooked
by mainstream society, there is a gap in understanding how racial and gender
discrimination, mixed-race cognitive dissonance, and sexual violence have
unique emotional repercussions for Indigenous peoples. One participant's
comments about school experiences and feeling oppressed when it came to
his Native American ancestry speak to the ways that external forces can impact
self-perception and vulnerability, affecting decision-making about issues like
obtaining therapy, dating, interacting with non-Native people, or in this case,
going to college:

> I hear everybody talking about their connection to their Native groups and
> for myself, you know, my father had always been the one to tell me, "Yeah,

you are, you are [Native]." And . . . you know, I went to [college]. And it just dawned on me now that I'm thinking, yeah, I've been having . . . have been, you know, oppressed all my life around my Native American origins. Um, it wasn't until I went to college that I was able to learn about my Native American culture and so I think I wanted to say . . . that you know, I think that there needs to be more education in the population at large. I mean you're asking about how do we get more people in [college]. Um . . . it's . . . people need to be educated, I believe, and you know, not oppressed. And to believe what people want them to believe [about themselves]. Because I do remember um . . . in elementary school where, you know, it's always supposed to be this certain way. And life isn't like that, you know, it's not the way it is. Um, it's just the way they wanted us to believe and to know. . . . But now after I had the chance to go to college, all these real issues have been brought to me and I have been able to go back to my culture. And it's through research and education that I'm able to know who I am as a person. We have to get people back in school, in college, to get the truth brought to them, you know. 'Cause most people don't make it to college.

This respondent's decision to attend college made an impact on how he came to address his feelings of being oppressed around his Native American culture. So while there was a high level of emotional risk in attending college, where Native people are in the minority, this person weighed the potential outcomes of this emotional risk and made positive strides toward healing from historical and intergenerational trauma. However, as the respondent also indicates, not everyone can make the same decision or have the same experience when it comes to attending a college or university. His statement speaks to why some Native people don't make the decision to attend college or to engage in other institutions that might reproduce feelings of oppression: to engage with these mainstream institutions can be a setup to reexperience painful emotional encounters with racism, sexism, and cultural bias.

In other cases, decision-making is determined not such much by emotion as by what I term a logic of vulnerability, which is connected to radical self-love. Some MLGBTQ2S participants made decisions very early in life that could be considered risky, but people who experience extremely high levels of trauma, violence, and mental abuse often find that the possibility of further marginalization no longer scares or threatens them. Potential positive outcomes are based on sentiments such as "What else can they do to me?" and "What else do I have to lose?"

When individuals feel that they no longer have anything to lose emotionally, physically, and/or financially, they are often willing to take risks that most within mainstream society would never consider, because daily interactions in mainstream society dictate that deviance from normalcy and stability is pathological. Living in a body constantly marked as aberrant, rapeable, and punishable leads to dehumanization—but these life experiences, when faced head on, can also lead to greater levels of subjectivity, self-determination, and transcendence. In other words, when we reject the negative ascriptions placed onto our bodies and experiences, we open up new possibilities for disidentifying and reworking definitions of ourselves that can be empowering rather than self-defeating (Muñoz 1999). Transgender participants spoke most vocally about taking pride in their bodies, often expressing profound levels of subjectivity and transcendence in their rejection of societal norms about who they should be and how they should live.

> And I left the house and like grew up in foster homes and residential treatment facilities, where I was, like, free to do what I want. So I started my transition, like growing my hair and wearing female clothes. And . . . I mean, I wasn't allowed to wear makeup but, I don't know . . . at the time I didn't really need it. I was young and everyone always thought I was a girl anyways. One time I was in juvie and these church people came and, like, preached to us in jail [speaker laughs]. And I'm like, "You're in the wrong cell." [Group laughs] They're like, "No I'm [sic] not." I just find that funny. . . . And another incident was like . . . um . . . these other church people came and the place where I was at, at the time, they have a gym and we were, like, throwing the football around, and I was, like, throwing the football. And they're like, "Damn, that girl has a good arm!" [Group laughs] I was like, I don't know . . . it just seemed like everyone was doing it. I was, like, trying to fool 'em and I always did too! Even when I'd go shopping, I'd always go in the men's room and they're like, "Oh sweetie you're going in the wrong one." And I'm like, "No I'm not!" And they're like, "Oh . . . well you're just a really pretty boy." And I was like, "Thanks . . ." So I don't know, it was just like that growing up.

This respondent, who also has a history of substance abuse and sexual violence, reveals a pattern, going back to childhood and adolescence, in which she consistently made decisions about her gender identity and her relationships with other people, including her family, based on what made her feel most comfortable. Despite having a troubled relationship with her father and facing the possible negative repercussions of beginning her transition at the age of thirteen, she made that choice anyway, not out of an emotional expectation or feeling, but as a form of differential consciousness, opposing normative behavior for a young boy and later for a young transgender person.[5] In another interview, this young woman described herself as doing what "I have to do," as a way of suggesting that despite all of the traumas and erasures she had experienced, she continued to believe that her own well-being and happiness were contingent on surviving. For her, that survival has frequently meant taking what others perceive as risks but that for her may not really be risks, because to live her life any other way would be a denial of who she is as a human being. She is aware that she could have been killed or seriously hurt along the way and yet, that possibility never stopped her from transcending the boundaries that society places in her way on a daily basis. She spoke more about these sentiments during one of our focus groups at NAAP:

> I started getting into drinking and smoking marijuana when I was kind of young, 'cause I moved back to the reservation after South Dakota. I mean South Dakota was good for me. I got a job and I worked a lot so I had money and I'd send it to my brother. I grew up with my brothers, we were always together so we were always close. And I guess . . . they found out . . . I mean, they didn't really care. They loved me for who I was and, you know, my mom found out as well. But she was kind of into drugs and drinking so, you know . . . she was never there either, growing up along with my dad. So it's like, my brothers were there for me. My mom didn't trip at all, she was like at first, "Oh what are you doing?" And I'm like, "Nothing. I'm doing what I want to do." And after that, it was kind of like whatever. And then, I don't know, I think I kind of look like her, so . . . I don't know, she just accepted it, like we got really close. And she's always like, "You're the daughter I never had." 'Cause I had four brothers. My dad was an asshole, I just never got in contact with him. And then I came here. . . . [I] wanted to go to school and start hormones and stuff. I mean I don't really need hormones 'cause I was really feminine. And I don't know, it was easy for me. I don't know why. I think it just . . . I believe God was, like, watching over me, kind of. There's a couple of instances where I'm pretty sure I could've died or something or . . . Obviously he's watching over me, you know.

The participant went on to mention that in states like Wyoming, because it is a bit more "New Age," people aren't really looking for "trannies or transgenders," unless they are attracted to transpeople. For transgender people, this participant believed, living in a "New Age" geographic location might mean having to face less scrutiny as an individual who falls outside heteronormative categories of identity. She also stated her belief that part of her success in blending in was because she had made the decision to live how she felt most comfortable; the examples from her two statements above demonstrate that others also saw her as cis-female, even before she had completed her transition.

The pathway to transcending sexual violence and experiences with sex work was not the same for all transgender participants. Another transgender participant who identifies as MTF (male to female) spoke about the roles that shame, Christianity, and emotional tension played when it came time for her to make decisions about how she self-identifies.

> I've always thought to myself, you know, what if I was born a girl, I wouldn't be running away from home. I wouldn't be coming out to my parents. I wouldn't be feeling this kind of loneliness. Like, to add onto it. I know exactly what it feels like not to have a gay friend because sometimes even in the communities we come from, you know, your friend's gay but hanging out with them is, like, even more, drawing attention. 'Cause, like, then you may have each other for support. But I knew if I was, if I was just a female I wouldn't be going through this. I wouldn't be suffering like this. But um . . . I guess on the racial thing, I knew that there was prejudice against Native Americans. But I didn't know to what extent. Until several years later, because I heard that . . . and this is probably not something I should have been told but when I started to distance myself from my family, one of the first things that they told me . . . and they come from a very Christian, conservative place in society . . . they told me that people had already forewarned them that Native Americans would kick you in the teeth if you tried to do anything good for them. Suddenly, you're like . . . You know, they would say that Native Americans are very unappreciative, very lazy, there was all these stereotypes associated with Indians. A lot of it was very hurtful. And I kind of never really sensed that my parents had had to stand up to racism with me. I never got that until several years later, when I was already an adult and we made our peace.

This respondent's desire to have been born a girl and to also have been born white, not a mixed-race Native American, speaks to the environmental context of trauma, mixed-race cognitive dissonance, gender discrimination, and sexual violence that MLGBTQ2S Natives face. Most people think of sexual violence as purely physical, but I would also argue that in the lives of many MLGBTQ2S people, sexual violence is also psychological. This transgender respondent, in contrast to the earlier participant, has white parents and did not grow up within a Native community, making it difficult for her to identify with being Native American. For this second respondent, making decisions did involve pausing to consider the emotional repercussions of identifying as American Indian and as female. Trauma, especially spirit-trauma, involves not only physical violence, but also includes forms of psychological violence that damage the well-being, self-esteem, and self-determination of victims in ways that often renders victims silent and mentally debilitated.

The divergence of experiences here is revealing. One participant was raised by Native parents who, despite being drug and alcohol users, still provided their child with an environment and cultural knowledge that made it possible for her to see her decision-making as a process for happiness, while the second participant, who received messages from family and others about how much easier life would be if she chose to be something else other than an Indian, sees her decision-making as a strategy to avoid emotional grief. By her own account, as the second participant began her transition to a new city, she learned the degree to which non-Natives would go to diminish and oppress Indigenous peoples:

> I did not know that I was, you know, unloved or that there was a whole genocide against my people. I really didn't. You know, I knew something had happened, and I knew it was unfortunate because when I came out to the city one of the first key things that I was told was, "Oh don't tell people you're Native American, don't tell people you're American Indian because they'll exploit you." Or "Change your name," they would tell me, "don't use your real name, get another name; be a different race." And that way you would be able to survive. There would be people apologizing to me, and I always felt awkward, you know, and for a while it was a little bit of my peeve because it was embarrassing that people would be saying, "I'm sorry [for] what happened to your people and I feel really terrible." Because they were white and I identified with white[ness] so easily because I was raised by a white and I didn't know anything but to be attracted to white men or to want to be a part of white society. I didn't go seeking Indians at that time, I went seeking white people and, you know, the social Christian churches and things like that. Things that had an association. . . . Like I said, I was always honest and forthcoming, so when I would tell people, "Oh I'm on my way to the city to become a prostitute," they would be like, "Oh no! We can't let you do that." So they would try to get me help and bring me to the city in Sacramento and they would even take me

themselves because I was such a young age. And I didn't know there was good
people. . . . 'Cause I was asking for money and there was people that were giving me money and then they weren't having sex with me. I always felt like I
was ripping them off. I just always wanted to be a beautiful female. I always
wanted to be a baby doll. I always wanted to be somebody's bitch. [Group
laughs] I did! There was years that I thought that maybe I shouldn't be coming out yet because there's just no money in the bank for pussy. For me to have
a pussy, you know [group laughter], so maybe I should just stay in the closet
and be gay for a while until I have enough money to pay for the whole thing.
But I didn't think along those lines, it was too easy to be myself. And I think
sometimes, you know, that's part of the joy of coming to a community like
this, that I was able to be myself. And have people care for me and love me for
my diversity.

This participant had felt isolated most of her life, living in a mostly white community and being raised by white parents, and it was not until she came to an
organization like NAAP that she finally felt loved and less afraid to embrace
all of her identities, all of her traumas—as well as to make decisions based not
on fear, but on her own love of self. As the final section of this chapter argues,
finding community and connections to spirituality, ceremony, and ancestors
can do a lot to address trauma, sexual violence, and colonial haunting in the
lives of MLGBTQ2S Natives. While this participant may have found strength
in meeting other Natives who identify with MLGBTQ2S characteristics, it is
important not to create a utopian view of Native-Native interactions. Many
of the acts of violence perpetrated against MLGBTQ2S people are committed
by older friends or relatives, creating mistrust between generations. This mistrust can prevent younger people from reaching out to older generations, with
their more "authentic" cultural knowledge, but there are always exceptions.
Some MLGBTQ2S people do have positive experiences of cross-generational
knowledge, acceptance, and community participation. Healing from violence
and trauma will require some degree of rebuilding trust between, across, and
within the multiple spaces and identities that occupy the lived experiences of
MLGBTQ2S people in contemporary urban environments.

ANCESTOR SPIRITS, CEREMONY, AND CULTURAL RECOVERY

One form of cultural resiliency exhibited by Indian Blood study participants in
the face of colonial haunting and marginalization stems from a deeply informed
connection to and understanding of tribal history, spirituality, ceremony, and

reverence for ancestor spirits. I define *ancestor spirits* as Indigenous relatives from previous generations who held particular forms of cultural and ceremonial knowledge that were effectively used in healing deeply held physical, spiritual, or emotional pain. These ancestor spirits reveal themselves to MLGBTQ2S Natives today through prayer, ceremony, and cultural practices that are tied to tribally specific memories, both precontact and postcontact, in the context of PTIS. As one participant described,

> I also think there's a purpose of me going to places like Oklahoma, when you are among people who are, like, richly involved with their traditional rituals. Um . . . they are different from the Indians who are involved in Christianity, or just the people who aren't involved in any sort of religious activity. I think those people who are involved in their, um, like the stomp dances and stuff are much less judgmental about things like me being gay or whatever. That really doesn't matter to them so much. It's more like, are you a good member of this community? You know, that's usually the hallmark of what the good person is, you know. And that's also my experience. Like, the women back there who are a part of the ceremonies, they accept me. They know that I'm gay and they could care less. . . . The guys are sometimes a little . . . But then they've been told by their elders that, that's, you know . . . They had to get over themselves.

Prayer and ceremony were important ways that participants were able to cope with sobriety issues related to drugs and alcohol. According to one participant, daily prayer and taking part in talking circles had increased his participation in the Native community and helped him in maintaining a more balanced life when it comes to health and the use of drugs and alcohol:

> My cultural identity was very always Native, very proud, Paiute. Instilled by my mom mostly because she wore the pants in the house. So our religious activity was [to] do our daily prayers, and I do that to this day religiously. That's part of my wellness dealing with diabetes. I'm HIV negative, but I work with a lot of AIDS clients and AIDS community [activists] and I've seen many challenges with their wellness as well. So I'm very proactive with the Native gay and lesbian community, Two-Spirit community now. And I just want to say I love San Francisco and I love our Native community. I do go to talking circles, I volunteer a lot. I'm very proactive and that's how I keep myself sober. I'm a binge drinker. I don't need alcohol everyday—not that type of person, but that is my use of drugs: alcohol.

This example speaks to the urban Indian context of practicing prayer, spirituality, and ceremony. For other participants, ceremony and social gatherings could also be important, depending on the context of the ceremony itself. Among members of the Native American Church, the use of peyote is not uncommon as a part of important individual and collective reflection, humility, vulnerability, and spiritual practice. However, the use of peyote for some MLGBTQ2S Natives also presents challenges when it comes to battling a history of abusing drugs and alcohol.

> I go to powwows . . . and some ceremonies, but others I really don't do anymore, like for instance, there was gonna be a . . . peyote ceremony one time, but I didn't go because if I were to take peyote, you know given my history . . . and the fact that everyone would be praying it would be difficult on me. And it would probably have a negative effect on me because you know, I used to, like, take LSD when I was a teenager and stuff. So I could go to certain ones [ceremonies] you know, but there are others where I wouldn't feel comfortable going.

The use of drugs and alcohol was a significant concern and factor in the health and wellness of participants. Survey responses reveal that many MLGBTQ2S participants had engaged in unprotected sex while using alcohol and drugs, making substance use a major risk factor for sexual violence and HIV transmission. While peyote was a concern for at least one participant, the overwhelming majority of participants spoke to the importance of reconnecting with ceremonial practice, especially if they had been unable to participate in ceremonies when they were growing up. Their responses reveal that participating in ceremony connects many MLGBTQ2S individuals to their ancestors, who experienced suffering through the initial stages of colonization. To connect with one's ancestor spirits helps to address intergenerational and historical traumas and provides a space for healing from sexual violence and other forms of oppression and marginalization. In fact, another participant spoke to the value of Native American peyote songs and traditions as a central aspect of his healing and reconnection with the diverse, mixed-Native community he grew up with in the Southwest:

> My family is from further south and we are very mixed, you know . . . We're the mixed, Mexica nation so . . . Um yeah it's been kinda interesting . . . I think that a lot of my friends growing up in school also identified in a similar way.

My friend who was from the reservation in El Paso, the Tewa Indians, is a
really good friend of mine and she was kind of my first introduction to Native
culture. Like, the Indigenous lifestyle was kind of foreign to me. . . . Like I
grew up, you know, Catholic school. That kind of thing. But I quickly . . . It
was like second nature to me, you know. We are still really good friends today.
I went to a peyote ceremony two years ago and now I'm thirty. And I go to do
the ceremony with her dad and a lot of my high school friends. And I thought
it was very interesting that, like, all of these kids that grew up like me, like,
not necessarily on a reservation or you know . . . identifying as Indians, that
we all grew up and we learned the peyote songs and the way of life. Even
though we weren't necessarily from that particular culture or whatever. It was
kind of neat to experience that as an older adult, like, looking back. . . . Like,
just the possibility of what all of us could have done. . . . It was really eye-
opening and heart-warming to go back to my hometown when I should have
had my high school reunion, like ten years after you graduate. To have actually had that and not had it be like a "school function" but to have it have been
just something that kind of naturally happened. And to have had it be a peyote
ceremony and to, like, have witnessed all my friends grown up and just, like,
taking to these traditions was really something powerful for me.

Here, we can observe the desire of MLGBTQ2S participants to connect with
their ancestors and living relatives through ceremony and traditions. These participants experienced contact with ancestor spirits as having the power to transform painful colonial memories and experiences into new decolonial moments
of cultural recovery and community revitalization. Transformative contact with
ancestor spirits is often realized through ceremonial spaces that renew the family and kinship ties broken during the process of Two-Spirit cultural dissolution
in the fifteenth and sixteenth centuries. As we have seen, the long history of
colonial assault against Native men, women, and children continues to produce tremendous inequalities and public health disparities. When you separate
a people from their cultural traditions and ways of knowing and supporting
one another, you produce powerful forms of what George Tinker describes as
cultural genocide (Tinker 1993). The Indian Blood participants, not unlike the
Native women who faced forced sterilization or the Indian children who suffered through sexual violence and corporeal punishment in boarding schools,
experience extreme spirit-traumas that reduce the possibilities for enacting
positive forms of agency, including radical love and ceremonial participation.
A return to participation in Native community practices, however, can support

MLGBTQ2S people in combating the historical and intergenerational traumas and stigmas that put them at greater risk for HIV.

Consider the following participant's comments about the correlation between his spiritual participation in ceremony and a positive sense of self-identity and community membership:

> I spent a lot of time traveling between here, San Francisco, and Austin, Texas growing up . . . um . . . And I got to spend a lot of time on reservations. I think that I found that it's kind of a spiritual or Native family. And I feel like a lot of questions that has [sic] been answered over the last couple of years. . . . Like, my identity is fulfilled. I think that I have come to a realization of who I am. I've always thought it's very interesting where like the Mexicans come from or the Lakota or the Hopi or the Tigua. . . . Like, how is it that they're truly recognized by other nations or other tribes, you know, as a true people. And I have been participating over the last ten years in a seven-year ceremony and I happened to show up, to just randomly show up for five of the seven years. And it was during that time that I guess I got to . . . when my ethnic, racial identity started to morph and as I try to call myself today I'm [Native name omitted for confidentiality] of the Rainbow nation. And that's who I really identify as and I try not to say that. It's not that I'm ashamed, but it's just you know, I want to avoid a hundred long questions. My name alone already is like telling somebody I got a puppy. You know, they're like "Are you Indian?" [speaker laughs] "Or did you have all your shots?" I just get all these questions and um . . . I, yeah, I've had a lot of really great experiences due to the connection with this ceremony. I've got to travel and change a lot because of it. And I think it's a big part of who I am now.

Ceremony allows many participants to rediscover cultural practices, traditions, and kinship support networks that were either inconsistent, absent, or hidden from them during their childhood and adolescence. The cultural recovery of spiritual practices takes place when individuals at high risk for HIV reconnect with the traumas of their ancestors and link those historical events with their own lived experiences, as cycles of intergenerational pain and abuse that can only be overcome through a reconnection to Indigenous ways of healing and living in contemporary society. Reconnecting with the historical traumas experienced by ancestors makes it possible to break the psychosocial patterns of internalized oppression and provides a means of achieving and building stronger kinship support networks. This reconnection is a process of radical love.

As this chapter has demonstrated, sexual violence is a significant factor in the life histories of MLGBTQ2S participants, but we have also observed the ways that a return to ceremony through connections with American Indian ancestors, elders, and spiritual leaders can mitigate some of the risks described by the IBPN risk model. There are still a number of important issues to consider when it comes to colonial haunting and its repercussions in an urban Indian context of discrimination based on gender, race, sexuality, and cultural practices. Chapter 7 takes up the issue of stress-coping strategies and practices within the context of racial mixing, public health disparities, and settler colonial projects that attempt to render Indians invisible. Social policies and economic competition continue to overlook, underfund, and shut down American Indian programming and culturally specific preventative health programs that could reduce the spread of HIV among MLGBTQ2S populations. Attaining the goal of decolonizing gender, sexuality, and mixed-race identity in the face of colonial haunting and HIV ultimately requires reconfiguring the separate and unequal status of American Indians as federally recognized nations, who should have the ability to determine which of their members are recognized and granted citizenship. These methods of granting citizenship must, however, deconstruct the ways that authenticity and validity are currently measured by Native nations, as a legacy of colonization that often reproduces the same inequalities that Native people have sought to address for so many centuries. In other words, decolonization must take urban Indians and mixed-blood identity into account not as obstacles to sovereignty and citizenship, but as necessary components of contemporary Indian identity. To fail to recognize urban, mixed-blood, and Two-Spirit identities is to fall into a pattern of internalized colonization that could mean the continuance of a policy of Native assimilation, reduction in population, and a bitter form of racism wielded no longer by non-Natives, but by Native peoples against themselves. As a community with 70 percent of its population living in urban areas and 70 percent of its population racially mixed, the Native community may have to "change its face" to preserve its existence.

CHAPTER 7

Stress Coping in Urban
Indian Kinship Networks

When I first came out to San Francisco, it was almost
a blessing in a way because I was always involved in Native
politics back in Oklahoma. But all of a sudden I didn't have
to be because nobody knew that I was [Native] anymore. So
I could just do my own thing. . . . But then all of a sudden I
started missing everything. And I think that's the wonderful
thing about this community out here in California.
Like, if you want to be connected back to the Native
community, it's very easy to do here.

—Indian Blood focus group respondent

FROM RELOCATION TO REUNIFICATION IN
THE MAKING OF THE URBAN INDIAN

The relocation program sponsored by the U.S. government began in the after-math of World War II, as American Indian veterans and others moved away from reservations and rural communities to larger metropolitan areas across the country (see Fixico 2000). Initially this was a voluntary migration, but by the early 1950s, it had expanded into a formal program. As Fixico explains, though it began as "an experiment to relocate employable Navajos to Denver, Salt Lake City, and Los Angeles, the program officially extended services to all qualified American Indians in 1952" (4). Like other migrating populations, those who were a part of the relocation program often found conditions in U.S. cities harsh, culturally foreign, and isolating. Building new relationships in these cities was not as easy as it might be today. The participant's comment that opens this chapter speaks to the experiences of being a Native mixed-blood, first in a reservation-based context, then in a large, urban setting like the San Francisco

Bay Area. As the respondent notes, he was initially happy to take a step back from Native identity politics, but he later found it easy to access Native organizations, events, and resources in the Bay Area. However, access to culturally specific resources has not always been readily available to those relocating to urban areas. Many who initially came could not find jobs, housing, or culturally specific resources to help them transition to the difficulties of living in a new, strange environment. Today, "the majority of the 2.1 million Indians live in cities" (Fixico 2000: 2). This shift in population density from reservation communities to urban environments caused yet another form of trauma for American Indian people, in much the same way that removal harmed the unity of Native families, clans, and kinship networks:

> The American Indian "family" found itself interrupted as loved ones migrated to the city. Sometimes they returned. American Indian men and women found their roles in life encountering drastic change from traditional outlooks to mainstream gender issues in a multicultural society. Wanting to find their tribespeople in cities, they sometimes grudgingly gave way to assimilation into the mainstream, compelling them to become "urban Indians" and to feel the sense of racism in a different way. Indian people faced a new reality as they clung to their identity, but many could not face it. These themes of individual person, family, gender, Native identity, race, cultural pluralism, assimilation, and urbanization involved American Indians and other people who experience life in American cities. (Fixico 2000: 3).

Urbanization, as Fixico describes, creates a new "generic Indian" identity in place of tribally specific identities. Here I want to argue that at present, more than sixty years since the beginning of the relocation program, the level of tribally specific knowledge and cultural practices passing from grandparent to parent and parent to child has eroded even further. However, as sociological theories in the field of migration studies propose, third-generation return among the grandchildren of participants in the relocation program is driving at least two aspects of American Indian urban identity today.[1] First, youth interest in tribally specific cultural programs and in returning "home" to the reservation in search of a deeper connection to tribal knowledge systems is on the rise, as more young people seek access to information that was denied their parents' generation.[2] Second, with the ongoing growth of the urban Indian population and the six-decade history of Native life in urban areas, urban re-creations and/ or co-creations of traditional tribal knowledge now constitute traditions of their own, which are both regionally and multi-tribal specific (Applegate Krouse 1999). These new traditional knowledge formations in cities like San Francisco are what I term traditional urban Indian cultural knowledge systems (TUICKS). TUICKS are unique organizational and community structures that govern a set of cultural protocols, practices, and collective investments that are particular to every distinct area of urban Indian relocation. The San Francisco Bay Area, for example, continues to organize itself around the Native American Health Center (NAHC), the Friendship House, powwows, and annual cultural events that are familiar to any long-term and accepted members of the urban Indian community (Lobo and Peters 2001). Members know one another. TUICKS provide them with a common language and a collective history that is the basis for the construction of urban Indian kinship networks. These networks can function in a traditional and culturally specific manner, in much the same way that reservations after removal were able to reconstitute the knowledge practices, ceremonies, and cultural protocols that are now seen as traditional to most reservations in the United States. Thus, TUICKS make it possible for multiracial identity to be one of many social markers that these urban Indian communities incorporate into an evolving and fluid definition of tradition. Furthermore, sexuality, gender, race, and even the concept of Two-Spiritedness may be not only tribally specific, but also TUICKS-specific.

For MLGBTQ2S individuals in the Bay Area, the incorporation of mixed-race identity as an assumed and semi-accepted aspect of the region's TUICKS opens up the possibility for more inclusion of MLGBTQ2S people in culturally specific programs, services, events, and organizations within this particular Native community. Over the six decades since the beginning of the relocation program, urban Indians have actively sought and found various forms of cultural reunification through their efforts to destabilize notions of there being a single Indian identity. In other words, as the urban American Indian community has become more diverse and more racially mixed, so too have they abandoned singular, essentialist notions of what it means to be an Indigenous person in the twenty-first century. While questions of authenticity remain central to Native politics in both rural and urban contexts, there has also been a shift in those racial politics as a result of changing demographics and a desire to preserve and maintain the American Indian community. As more Native people experience racial mixing and cultural change over time, once-rigid definitions of what it means to be Native are broadening, in a move toward self-preservation. While questions of Indian "authenticity" persist, they are also more regularly debated, contested, and reconfigured (Garroutte 2002, Sturm 2002, Jolivette 2007,

Barker 2012, Klopotek 2011). For urban Indians in general, and for MLGBTQ2S Indians in particular, the sooner individuals refrain from chasing an illusory "essential" Indian identity, the more access they will have to urban-Indigenous stress-coping mechanisms and TUICKS that can reduce the pressures noted in the IBPN model, and in the process reduce the risk for HIV transmission.

TOWARD URBAN-INDIGENOUS STRESS-COPING MECHANISMS

Indigenous stress-coping mechanisms have been shown to reduce the effects of colonization and by extension, to mitigate the psychological and social problems that lead to high-risk sexual behavior and HIV transmission among MLGBTQ2S Natives.[3] In their seminal essay outlining an "indigenist" stress-coping model for American Indian women, coauthors Karina Walters and Jane Simoni (2002) examine the ways that cultural factors mitigate risk and act as buffers that strengthen psychological and emotional health. MLGBTQ2S participants are seeing an increase in their participation in TUICKS through their peer relationships with other MLGBTQ2S people and through their growing access to American Indian-specific organizations such as NAAP, BAAITS, and NAHC, all located in the San Francisco Bay Area. These organizations and other Native-specific groups across the nation are linked by their culturally specific focus in rendering health care services. In the context of the San Francisco Bay Area, stress-coping becomes crucial for many Natives who are away from family and friends and need support in order to enact their safer sex intentions. The formation of what I term TUICKS is akin to what Renya Ramirez terms Native hubs:

> In addition, many participate in what we might call virtual hubs, instances when hub-making occurs without a specified location or any formal organization. This kind of hub-making interaction might include a grandmother telling stories about her childhood on the reservation to her grandchildren, or one Native youth talking to another about visits to a tribal land base. This other kind of less formal Native hub, this hub as concept and process rather than geographic place or organization has a potential effect—encouraging young people to *imagine* a tribal homeland, thereby strengthening a rooted connection to tribe and tribal identity. (171–72)

These Native hubs, like TUICKS, rely not on place so much as on people in Indigenous communities with the capacity to share experiences that re-create feelings of home, support, and belonging. These new spaces create buffers against stress for MLGBTQ2S Natives in the San Francisco Bay Area.

One participant shared his experiences with stress and how, despite challenges, he has begun a healing process as a result of his participation within the San Francisco Native community. His quote below includes three important points. First, it was through another mixed-blood Native that he was able to identify Native-specific organizations to help him address difficulties he was having with sobriety, post-incarceration anxiety, and health services. Having a counselor who is also of mixed-race Native ancestry provides an added level of comfort for MLGBTQ2S participants like this one; MLGBTQ2S people often face doubts about their ability to access services, because of their mixed-race backgrounds. Having another mixed-race Native recommend Native-specific services allowed this young man to feel that his identity would not be a problem. Second, the quote underscores the importance of ethnic-specific organizations as central units of a new, urban Indian kinship network. Third, the participant's emphasis on shared activities and community support demonstrates that urban Indian kinship networks at their foundation are supported and maintained by TUICKS:

> Well I first came to the Native American AIDS Project in 2001. And I was seeking substance abuse [help]. . . . I had been recently incarcerated and I was um . . . After my incarceration, I started coming out on the street with this new attitude of like, "Oh it could happen again, I could get put in jail again. I could be in trouble if I don't stop, if something doesn't change." So I was looking around and I . . . through the Delancey Street, one of the counselors that was partially Native, and when I told him about my um . . . what my ethnicity was, 'cause I've always identified as American Indian, he referred me to Native American AIDS Project. And I came over here for their harm reduction services and for their peer counseling. They had a wonderful program back then that had involved groups and talking circles and just wonderful bead classes through the Native American Health Project, that I met other people at. And I really needed this because I came out of . . . I came up from really knowing nothing but . . . that there . . . that there . . . the raw idea that I've got to somehow make it. So I went down to the General Assistance Office with Social Services. And I applied for the GA, which I had never done before. I never knew anything about GA because I had always provided [for] myself through prostitution. I had always somehow struggled and scrapped to get by, you know. Until I got incarcerated I had no idea that I couldn't do it forever.

Navigating the complexities of urban life presents many MLGBTQ2S people with enormous challenges. Many have never lived off the reservation; for others, simply understanding the resources available to them is a major challenge, as most health, employment, and government services are complex and written in ways that the general population cannot easily negotiate. For example, despite the passage of the Affordable Care Act under President Obama, nearly 23 million people will continue to live without health insurance (Vestal 2013). The majority of these people will come from poor communities, Indigenous communities, and communities of color across the country. Several thousand will not understand how to sign up for the new health exchanges, while others simply won't qualify because they will not meet "poverty requirements" to qualify through Medicaid and Medicare. Ethnic-specific organizations such as NAAP and BAAITS not only provide an urban Indian kinship network for health services, they also strengthen cultural connections that enhance stress-coping mechanisms among MLGBTQ2S populations.

Participants reported that urban Indian kinship networks helped them not only in accessing health care, but also in obtaining both cultural knowledge and cultural capital. One MLGBTQ2S participant described how support from peers at NAAP allowed him to find his way to other social services that made it possible to refrain from returning to his previous work in prostitution:

> I came here and I met wonderful people, they referred me to BAAITS. I started drumming and I just . . . As things got better for me, I wanted to . . . you know, be a part of it. But as things got better for me, other things came into my life that I had no idea what to do. . . . So I guess now . . . I mean things are so much better than where I was. My stress levels as a child were high because there was no . . . there was nothing to fall back on. You either go out there and did it, stress or not, you know. A little bit of acne has never stopped nobody from getting their money right? [Group laughs] So I would get out there and do it, but it's nice to be able to just sit back and take a breather and know that I can work through these moments where I feel bad. And I can turn to other people. And I can turn to this group [at NAAP]. And I can turn to groups like this one too [the Indian Blood focus group] . . . to heal myself. Because this actually is a healing for me. And this is wonderful because I don't get to enjoy as much since I moved further away.

It is significant that this participant found a familial type of support and kinship, not during his childhood but as an adult, and within an urban Indian context.

His mention of the focus group as a place where he could turn also speaks to the comfort he felt in discussing his struggles with incarceration, prostitution, and sobriety with other individuals from similar backgrounds. Other participants agreed that they saw value in having a specific space to address health, wellness, and healing with other people of mixed-race Native ancestry and through MLGBTQ2S-specific services and organizations.

That the participants spoke to the importance of ethnic-specific and culturally competent health services as vital safety nets in HIV prevention should come as no surprise. Research literature in the field of HIV over the past twenty years suggests strong links between cultural influences and HIV risk.[4] Because these links have been made, many public health providers and researchers continue to call on health care and social service workers to take culture into account when planning, implementing, and evaluating HIV prevention programs. There is also a need for greater levels of support for developing effective protective factors within communities of color. Protective factors are particularly important in the assessment of successful prevention programs. In the San Francisco Bay Area, besides NAAP, the only other ethnic-specific organizations that cater to the needs of Indigenous peoples are NAHC, BAAITS, and the Asian Pacific Islander (API) Wellness Center. Mainstream health organizations and HMOs often lack a focus on the broad societal-level forces (i.e., poverty, racism, sexism, homophobia, transphobia) that weaken both individual protective factors and community-based beliefs, attitudes, and norms about gender roles, as well as about cultural differences in communication among sexual partners and health providers (Solomon, Berman, and Card 2007). Decisions about dating and intimate sexual relationships also have a bearing on stress levels and coping mechanisms. One participant was forthcoming in stating that she did not have the best coping mechanisms, but implies that while she takes out her frustrations on her partner, she is able to process these actions and is looking for healthier ways to address the problems in her life:

> I have my partner now and I guess I don't really deal with stress well. Often times I'll react, I'll react out of hurt or frustration, or sometimes just out of selfishness. And I just have to say that I'm really fortunate to have a realization later after the fact of what I'd spewed or whatever I've been up to. And then I can come back and I can say, "Oh gosh! I'm so sorry that this happened." Or you know, it just really felt good to get it off my chest but I don't feel good with the consequences. I don't feel good that people are now looking at me [as] someone who can't hold their alcohol or maybe like . . . maybe I should stop

being such a bitch! But um . . . as far as stress, you know, when I have stress I think I've always been that kind of person that would rather run away from stress than have to deal with it. So I'm a little bit . . . I'm still learning to deal with stress. I like music, I like dance. I'm not as stressed as I used to be.

This participant, like others, has worked very hard to reduce stress and find positive ways to deal with her emotional triggers. Native-specific organizations, despite having limited resources, are assisting MLGBTQ2S people by creating a family environment where individuals from this population can work together to reassess past patterns and behaviors. Often, these Native-specific grass-roots organizations like NAAP and BAAITS do not have the infrastructure or resources to maintain their daily operations as mainstream organizations and hospitals do, and they are often forced into competing for resources with other ethnic-specific organizations like API Wellness Center, Friendship House, and NAHC. One participant, a transgender woman, spoke to how these grassroots organizations not only provide culturally competent HIV prevention services, but also create a family environment based on kinship, where every individual is valued as part of a larger community, fostering a larger urban Indian kinship network of support and resiliency.

I want to come home and be able to be . . . you know, happy. To have my sisterhood. 'Cause growing up there was a lot of prostitutes like me and we all had a connection. And it was, just immediately, [we] became like family. Um . . . geez . . . Where am I going to go if there's no Native American AIDS Project? I don't know . . . Right now I'm just so happy to be able to volunteer my time here and I know that BAAITS has done so much work to keep these grassroots organizations afloat. So you know, without these things, things are gonna be a little bit harder. We're gonna have to rely on the people that we know I guess, the contacts and the emails, it's still very new to me. But if I can stay in the loop then I'll sign up for any kind of emails. Just to be a part of it, even though I'm so far away now. It's really nice to go to powwows. It's nice to be involved. It's nice to have people remember my name and to have seen so many people for so many years and . . . I just love being Indian! And so it's nice to have other people out there that love being Indian and gay and trans, and . . . all that!

These comments suggest a high degree of self-acceptance and a developed ability to be emotionally vulnerable with others. This participant has been through many challenges in her life and yet does not "feel bad" about herself or her body. She also speaks to the importance of urban Indian kinship networks in providing her with support she needs to continue to live a healthy life, even in the face of discrimination and abuse. Before she came to NAAP she had experienced extreme levels of sexual violence that took a tremendous toll on her, but as her statement above suggests, she has made a lot of progress toward healing because of her participation in Native-specific organizations. Her comments below reveal how different life was before she came to NAAP for services:

> Back then [government assistance] was my lifeline. You know, it really did keep me out of trouble. And it didn't really do a very good job of that, because I'd always find a little bit of something to get into. But that was part of it, you know. And as far as dating, yeah! I really felt bad for all the people that statutory raped me, but I don't feel bad for myself. I don't feel bad about my body. I knew about the HIV crisis. I came out as a part of it. I knew about condoms, I knew about being a stickler. You know, like the young lady here said, I must have had a really good angel. Or a really good source because I never had any problem praying for what I needed. And I remember myself praying every night before I'd step out there in them heels, I'd be like, "Give me a good one tonight! I want to make two hundred dollars like the last girl. I want to avoid being arrested; I want to come home without HIV."

Before coming to NAAP, this participant relied heavily on non-Native sources of support and turned toward sex work and high-risk behaviors to cope with ongoing experiences with colonial trauma. Her identity as a transgender MTF person, coupled with her mixed-race background, also suggests the salience of identity categories in the shaping of emotional, physical, and spiritual well-being among MLGBTQ2S people in the San Francisco urban Indian community.

Identity, as we have seen, plays a major role in the resiliency of MLGBTQ2S people, and mixed-race identity, according to many of the focus group respondents, does impact the strength of urban Indian kinship networks. For instance, some participants felt that the Native community in the Bay Area was sufficiently accepting that there was no need for services tailored to mixed-race Natives, while others believed that addressing the persistence of discrimination based on racial identity for mixed bloods would only strengthen culturally responsive prevention programs and cultural support networks. One participant said,

I don't think there's too much of a mixed-race community, but, um, I think there's a lot of people that are mixed, that maybe should have, uh, a chance to talk about it. I mean . . . and it probably, what they would do, is make groups, kind of like AA groups . . . like they could have a big building and they could have certain kinds of groups there going on, and maybe it would be good to try to get one going in this town or somewhere one of these days. I think people still look down on someone if they want to, have hatred toward somebody and they can always pick something like, mixed-race, or gender, or whatever they want. I think that stems from prejudice and not just hate. They just, um, feel superior to somebody and have control issues, stuff like that.

Developing what I would term a critical mixed-race community ethic of health and wellness must include a deep commitment to cultural competence. MLGBTQ2S participants see the value of both American Indian and mixed-race specific mental health programs. These types of programs, however, can only prove successful if they include what public health interventionists term the "building blocks of cultural competence." According to Solomon, Berman, and Card (2007), "building culturally competent HIV prevention programs involves the culturally related needs of program participants" (8). They argue that doing this work in an effective and sustained manner requires four factors. The first is looking inward "at agency and staff norms, values, beliefs, and assumptions." For MLGBTQ2S participants, this means that agencies like NAAP, NAHC, BAAITS, and others that serve this community must constantly reassess how their staff values and beliefs differentially impact MLGBTQ2S people. In the second element, looking outward "at how cultural factors affect HIV-related behaviors and access to and use of services," health care providers must also work to get to know their clients as people and not simply as patients. Looking outward entails the active and conscious reevaluation of current program models that seek to address HIV-related stress factors and stigmas such as those detailed in the IBPN model. In chapter 8, I take up this issue of program needs and intervention model reevaluation to suggest possible approaches that organizations like the NAHC might undertake to meet the specific needs of MLGBTQ2S populations who are risk for HIV infection. In Solomon, Berman, and Card's third element, applying knowledge, hospitals and health agencies working with populations like MLBGTQ2s should "apply knowledge to HIV prevention programming in ways that address cultural factors relevant to HIV prevention." Finally, building the blocks of cultural competence requires facilitating a process of "actively involving clients in planning, implementation, evaluation processes and treating them with respect and sensitivity."

These four steps are also central to creating successful strategies for decolonizing gender, sexuality, and mixed-race identity. In particular, the fourth element of building cultural competence asserts that clients need to be involved in planning, implementation, and evaluation processes. This step ensures that the subjectivities of MLGBTQ2S people are at the center, not the margin. Decolonizing gender, sexuality, and mixed-race identity in the face of colonial haunting and HIV requires deconstructing and transforming colonial representations, policies, and positions of power while also empowering both new and old Indigenous cultural knowledge systems, which have their own distinct and diverse ways of understanding gender, sexuality, and race. Healing from the aftermath of Two-Spirit cultural dissolution also means understanding that the Western construction of "the" Native as a singular, fixed, already raced, sexed, and gendered body must be abandoned in favor of Indigenous-centered approaches to inclusivity, positive stress-coping, and an increase in intergenerational healing and leadership across generations.

STRESS-COPING, DATING, AND RESILIENCY FACTORS

In their statements, *Indian Blood* participants reveal how factors such as gender, colorism, and racial objectification impact their everyday choices, from obtaining services at Native-specific organizations to selecting intimate dating and/or sexual partners. Many of the comments by MLGBTQ2S Natives in the San Francisco Bay Area suggest that colonial trauma creates divisions within the American Indian community and causes some individuals to feel unsafe when it comes to privacy, disclosure, and the strategies they utilize to address HIV status, social stigmas, and activities that foster resiliency. One participant, who is active in HIV and sexual health education work, recounts how his HIV diagnosis leads to feelings of isolation. His comments also suggest that engaging with Native-specific groups, organizations, and activities helped him to find his own unique set of stress-coping strategies. These strategies, like those utilized by other MLGBTQ2S Natives, led to greater levels of resiliency in the face of colonial trauma and HIV risk:

> I have primary care through my job, so if I need medical services, I just go to
> Kaiser. Um . . . they also offer, like, counseling services. For example like, um
> . . . when I seroconverted, which was a very big momentous thing, one thing

I didn't do, was I didn't want to come to NAAP. Because I was sort of embarrassed. I was working in this field for a long time, and then to seroconvert
means that I like didn't take any of the lessons that I knew in my head were
the safe sex practices to protect myself. And I didn't follow those. I wasn't
walking the path. I wasn't like, um . . . walking the talk. Um . . . and . . . so I
didn't come here—I also didn't come here 'cause I didn't feel that it necessarily reflected who I was. Um . . . I felt, like, the staff was mostly women, and I
wanted to see a gay Indian guy here. And that didn't really happen here for
me. I was—they might be here, but it wasn't my impression of the staff. And I
would have preferred to have that be the case. Um . . . I guess um, hmm . . . I
am very involved with, like, a gay Native drag group. So we do a lot of expres-
sive things that, express a lot of emotion, and that sort of creative acting
aspect allows you to get a lot of . . . allows you to express a lot of things, you
know, in a different way. And I think that always helps me. Um . . . and then
I'm pretty close with my two older brothers, so I can basically tell them anything. Um . . . and I'm pretty close with my family. And I'm totally out to them.

It is of interest to note that this participant specifically sought mainstream
services after his seroconversion because he was embarrassed to have other
Natives who work in the field find out that he had become HIV positive. He also
points out that he sought a particular connection based on gender, an aspect
of identity that he didn't immediately see at NAAP. As his story demonstrates,
MLGBTQ2S people often find it difficult to access stress-coping and resiliency
strategies, which colonial trauma can put out of reach by making it difficult
for members of this Native demographic to connect with their own communities out of fear of rejection or judgment. The quote also highlights the ways
that affinities, including those of gender, race, and sexuality, are of paramount
importance to marginalized populations who are at risk for or already living
with HIV or other illnesses (Diaz 1997).

Gender identity was not the only concern voiced by MLGBTQ2S participants
in relation to effective stress-coping and resiliency factors. Others spoke quite
candidly about colorism and racial objectification as challenges in dating that
could lead to high-risk sexual behavior if not addressed in a routine, positive
manner. All of these forms of objectification are adding to stress levels among
MLGBTQ2S Natives, who, by virtue of the their varied and blended social and
cultural identities, experience multiple layers of subtle and not-so-subtle doubts
about being accepted by friends, colleagues, and perhaps most importantly by
potential intimate partners. One participant who grew up identifying as a gay

male shared his experience of making the transition from gay male to transgender female and described how both gender and race factor into the ways that she is coming to understand and accept herself as a MLGBTQ2S person in the broader urban Indian community of the San Francisco Bay Area:

> My experience . . . wow. My experience like I said before as a gay man, was totally different. Like the dating scene, and my exes, ex-boyfriends . . . it was totally different. Um, I was younger then, now I'm in a relationship . . . and it's been three months, four months, and it's been up and down, up and down. It's my first transgender relationship. And it's very uncomfortable for me sometimes, because when you start out to bring transgender [identity in], you're already subconscious about everything, then to be in a house with someone and take your showers or baths or to get dressed, stuff like that, it's difficult. Especially if you're starting out, you're still kind of like a queen, you're not really transgender, you know what I mean? There is a difference, you know what I mean? And just because you've been on hormones a couple of months does not make you a TS, at all. It doesn't, though and I know for a fact, I mean, it doesn't. 'Cause I have a lot of tendencies and stuff like that, and my dating habits are like still like a gay boy instead, instead of being a transgender woman. You know, so it's like the longer—um, because like I said he's my first boyfriend since I started my life as being transgender—the longer we're in that relationship, the more I learn about being a transgender woman, though. . . . And it kind of really helps though, when you, when you're in a relationship—because you are like, it's your experience for the first time, it's like, what you are gonna be? . . . I don't know how to explain this, um . . . how do I explain that? Um . . . it's new. You know what I mean though, and it's, like, teaching me.

Gender identity is complex and fluid, and differs for every individual. That this one person doesn't feel like a transgender woman yet because she has not been in a relationship as a transgender person is only one perspective on transgender identification. And yet her comments underscore the subconscious and conscious ways that gender constructions can force individuals to feel trapped by gender binaries constructed during the colonial period. This same participant went on to discuss how being transgender, like any gender identity, is a constantly evolving process and that one learns by engaging in new and different experiences—including struggles to decolonize gender, sexuality, and race in contemporary society—that shape a sense of self.

You know, it *is* though [teaching me]. Regardless of, like . . . [I'm] totally not in a perfect relationship, but it's not terrible either. But it's just, like it's teaching me though, and it's letting me learn, and it's just like a totally different life for me. Even, you know, before I met him being single transgender, or queen, I was, but um . . . it's different, having dates or having a boyfriend, it's totally different. And, um, it's just a learning experience though, and . . . so my experiences have been just totally different though, like I said, you know . . . I have been an object though, and I had a lot of people dating me because of my skin color. Not so much the race, but the complexion of your skin. 'Cause it's fair, not fair, but it's kind of light, or light brown or whatever. Um, I've had a lot of that, though, being, you know, mixed-race and all . . . not so much the race though, because it's the color, because you can be mixed with some things and you can be dark or light, or in between, you know what I mean though? And I've had my experiences and some have been because of the color, and stuff, and um . . . It bothers me, though, and um, it does bother me, though. He is one of the first people I've dated, though, that—he didn't really care about what color I was. He doesn't care, you know, and . . . it's like, whether I'm short hair, long hair, blond, black, blue, whatever . . . he, you know, he doesn't really care. So that's a good thing.

As this participant's experience illustrates, dating and the development of intimate sexual relationships have the potential to deeply impact stress-coping, protective factors, and resiliency among populations that are vulnerable for HIV infection. In fact, when we consider the IBPN risk model factors (Two-Spirit cultural dissolution, historical and intergenerational trauma, racial and gender discrimination, mixed-race cognitive dissonance, and sexual violence) and examine their impact on dating patterns we can identify a positive correlation between higher rates of unprotected anal intercourse and stress-coping avoidance (Martin, Pryce, and Leeper 2005). Fostering positive, intimate relationships, along with friendships and community support networks, can produce environments that sustain mutual accountability, resiliency, and reciprocity.

In the face of more than five hundred years of colonial narratives that limit the possibilities for Indigenous-defined categories of gender, race, and sexuality, decolonization of these categories will require a consistent and collective effort to reshape the lenses that Native people use to understand themselves, with the help of their own ontological frameworks. The word decolonization has become quite popular over the last several decades and I do not use it here lightly. Decolonization will take many years, perhaps many generations, to accomplish: where does this leave populations like MLGBTQ2S Natives, who are today facing multiple forms of colonial marginalization within the context of the HIV epidemic? Ceremony and community healing can restore on a daily basis the deep social and psychological damage caused by ongoing settler colonialism and colonial haunting, in effect destabilizing the archaeologies of gender, sexuality, and race that limit the unique, diverse, and ever-changing landscape of indigeneity in urban areas. MLGBTQ2S populations demand and deserve greater cross-generational dialogue, support, and mentoring programs that are specific to ethnicity, gender, and sexuality.

Organizations like NAAP provided this type of support and yet, when these organizations are no longer able to keep their doors open, stress and discrimination become primary determinants of high-risk sexual behavior. In cases like these, when organizations do not have the capacity to meet the needs of all of their clients, urban Indian kinship networks of support become a secondary safety net. TUICKS should therefore include processes for peer mentoring and positive relationship-building, in order to rebuild a Two-Spirit ethic of support and communal healing after years of mistrust within marginalized groups. Western models of psychotherapy do not meet the needs of many MLGBTQ2S people because often "the/rapists" make clients feel like they are being re-victimized. Instead, as participating members in the formation of TUICKS, many MLGBTQ2S Natives in the Bay Area rely on new, urban Indian kinship networks that include not just blood kin, but also friends and mentors who often act as surrogate families who can support positive changes in behavior that promote health and wellness. As one participant said, "I used to go to the therapist, but now, I go visit my friends, mostly just for support because of what's going on with my life. I have to tell somebody what's going on with my life. . . . I have friends I can call up and just talk and ask them what their opinion might be. . . . I could relate more to my friends than a therapist. I don't want to tell [therapists] all the dirty, dirty things, you know. I just tell my friends and there's always support there."

Relationality in these instances is an important aspect of decolonizing gender, sexuality, and mixed-race identity. In an ideal situation, MLGBTQ2S populations would have strong relationships where they could talk openly and vulnerably with therapists, doctors, teachers, and other social service professionals, but falling short of this they need to have a secondary level of support from friends, family, and community members. The greatest blow struck by colonization continues to be the internalization of non-Native views of race, gender, and sexuality. Thus, decolonization requires the reacquisition of the power to name and create Indigenous communities, in particular through an inclusive ecological sovereignty (IES) model (described in chapter 4). The life stories of MLGBTQ2S American Indians in the San Francisco Bay area offers a compelling case study of the importance of decolonization as a public health concern in the lives of Indigenous peoples in the Americas and the Pacific. Intergenerational healing and cultural leadership programs can (if institutionalized within ethnic-specific organizations) potentially reduce high levels of trauma, stress, and risky sexual behavior. This book's final chapter offers an intervention model to address issues of decolonization, positive stress-coping, and MLGBTQ2S healing through leadership activities and engagement with other MLGBTQ2S American Indians.

CHAPTER 8

Two-Spirit Return

Intergenerational Healing
and Cultural Leadership among
Mixed-Race American Indians

I mostly turn to my friends. . . . I do a couple
different things every year. I go to Oklahoma, go to
ceremonies. I'm very involved with the local Cherokee
community. I've been asked [by the] Cherokee Nation to do
community organizing for San Francisco and the Bay Area.
So I've recently went through a leadership training.
I got sent back to Oklahoma to do leadership training
and share what I've learned here [in the Bay Area]
with folks back home on the reservation.

—Indian Blood focus group respondent

INDIGENOUS CULTURAL MENTORING NETWORKS

INDIGENOUS CULTURAL MENTORING NETWORKS (ICMNS) OFFER
counterhegemonic models for improving stress-coping mechanisms while
simultaneously reducing high-risk behaviors among MLGBTQ2S populations
in the San Francisco Bay Area. These models not only have the potential to
increase positive stress-coping measures in the face of colonial trauma, but
they also present tangible strategies and interventions that can reduce rates of
HIV infection among this population. ICMNs can also serve as mechanisms to
achieve decolonization and Two-Spirit return. Striving for Two-Spirit return,
however, entails an acceptance of the regionally specific context of the term
Two-Spirit, as created, maintained, and practiced within the TUICKS of the
San Francisco Bay Area and other places where Indigenous peoples re-create

American Indian communities outside their original tribal homelands. The term Two-Spirit, as discussed throughout this book, is not a fixed, universal category that can be applied to all American Indian tribes and nations. However within TUICKS, Two-Spirit return can and should include a process for self-determination and self-definition articulated by MLGBTQ2S people who, together with other Indigenous people, can engage in urban Indian kinship networks. Such networks can, in combination with IES models, bring together all of the diverse peoples that make up the American Indian and Alaskan Native population of the United States.

Many *Indian Blood* participants spoke to the need for stronger kinship networks that include local Native friends with shared identities, as well as a need for balance between these urban networks and ceremony within their respective nations. The quotation that opens this chapter raises important and fundamental questions about leadership, ceremony, and reciprocity as mechanisms for healing within the American Indian community. While there are very few studies that assess the efficacy of peer-mentoring programs in reducing high-risk sexual behavior, one study has demonstrated that peer mentoring interventions can mitigate rates of injection drug use and other high-risk behaviors associated with HIV seroconversion (Purcell, Metsch, Latka, Santibanez, Gomez, Eldred, and Latkin 2007). Purcell and his coauthors combined multiple influences in developing their intervention, including social learning theory, empowerment, and peer leadership or advocacy. In the intervention, "participants were told . . . that we wanted to help them try out a new social role as informal peer mentors and that learning this role would help them to protect themselves and their communities (using the slogan "power to protect")" (S113). Their success suggests that programs designed along these lines can be effective in both disease management and prevention among marginalized groups.

The peer mentoring program developed by Purcell and his coauthors for injection drug users provides some insight into possible ways to organize peer mentoring interventions aimed at reducing the transmission of HIV in MLGBTQ2S populations. Modifications to Purcell's model should consider the priority concerns of MLGBTQ2S Natives, incorporate cultural knowledge, and create a scale to measure and address both historical and intergenerational trauma, as well as existing stress-coping mechanisms, in order to ensure that such interventions are effective within this specific population. The Purcell model relies quite heavily on traditional Western approaches to mentoring and prosocial behavior, and does not explicitly consider the ramifications of psychosocial trauma on populations that experience PTIS. An effective and responsible approach to peer mentoring among Indigenous peoples must emphasize cultural knowledge, harm reduction, and community leadership through social and political participation.

Many MLGBTQ2S respondents spoke to their experiences with revictimization and weak health and wellness networks. The fear of revictimization coupled with fragile health support networks gives many vulnerable populations pause about participating in new studies, including interventions like these. Consider the following statements made by *Indian Blood* participants:

I couldn't tell you, besides my brother . . . I couldn't tell you any of my brothers' and sisters' birthdays. I don't know them. I don't keep those kinds of things in my brain. But um . . . yeah, it's as if we're going to doctors and stuff regularly. . . . It's only recently that I've actually needed to go to the doctor, and it's like, I didn't know where to go. I don't have the money. I don't have insurance. So I was like, where am I gonna go? But I'm not enrolled, so I was like, can I go to the Indian Health Center? Will they take me? Or Valley Medical, where they'll just charge you later . . . lots and lots of money! But it was like, hmmm, no, I've always just muddled through, like my boss says about me, "I don't know how you always do it, you just keep marching on!" It's like, well there's not too many other choices. You either just lay down and die or keep going. And I keep going, usually with a smile on my face.

Uh . . . I don't know . . . I actually . . . the last time I saw a doctor it was retraumatizing. It was at the health center. He wanted to do a genital examination, and I said, "I have a history of sexual abuse. Absolutely not!" When I'm down on the table, he does what he wants to do. And when I brought it up with the health center, then it's . . . victimize, or revictimize, or . . . blame the victim type, type of thing. After that point, it's just, you know, what it is. . . . No matter where you go, it's Western medicine. . . . It's a long history of abuse, um, and until it really approaches a position of holistic care, then I might consider it. But I deal with what—I deal with that a lot and, um, I just keep going. And I do get a lot of lectures, but ironically a lot of women understand why I refuse services. 'Cause I'm not . . . You know, I did the adult thing, I did the "right" thing and yet even though I went and done what was suppose to be the "right" thing, it like, um . . . Don't disempower me! 'Cause that could be deadly at some point, more so for the other side.

These responses not only speak to the ongoing challenges of policing Indian identity for those who are mixed-blood and/or unenrolled, they also demonstrate that many people in the Native community of the San Francisco Bay Area are struggling to just "keep going on" with few health care options. While the recent expansion of Medicare under the Affordable Care Act promises to benefit millions of more Americans, American Indians have historically rejected free U.S. government-sponsored health programs, including Indian Health Services, so it is unclear if, without targeted and culturally specific outreach strategies, there will be any increase in the number of Native people enrolling in Medicare programs. The participants' quotes also demonstrate this mistrust through their condemnation of the fact that even within some Native-specific organizations, there may be doctors and non-Native staff who treat patients with the same kind of care that they might receive from nonethnic-specific hospitals. As the second participant pointed out, he doesn't want to feel disempowered or revictimized as a survivor of sexual violence.

So how do we address the needs of MLGBTQ2S populations within the context of ongoing colonial medical practices? At least two steps are essential to developing a peer mentoring intervention model, or any intervention, for MLGBTQ2S Natives. First, it is important to structure interventions that consider ethnic, tribal, and cultural affinity. While there can be some possible drawbacks to this—because many of the factors associated with the IBPN model can be retraced back to tribal communities of origin or families, causing distrust between younger and elder generations or between those who share particular ethnic, gender, or sexual orientation affinities—it is still important that MLGBTQ2S individuals be paired with mentors who have a similar background and experience, if we are to expect intervention participants to feel safe sharing their stories and experiences. Second, both mainstream and ethnic-specific health organizations must consider how they lack the infrastructure to support ethnic, gender, and culturally specific peer mentoring groups. HIV support groups or prevention models within mainstream hospitals do not meet the cultural competence needs of many MLGBTQ2S people, nor do these facilities consider the impact of white racism within queer communities as potentially destructive to peer mentoring that is interracial. One participant spoke of his experience with Kaiser's HIV support group and how whiteness and the fear of white sexually predatory behavior impacted his choices in selecting a peer support group in the Bay Area:

> Kaiser has two HIV support groups, and it had, like, a gay men's group and, like, a mixed group of people. And I decided, after I heard things about both groups, that I really didn't want to go to the gay one because I felt that it was mostly an older, long-term survivor sort of group, of mostly gay white men.

And I just felt I didn't, I wasn't going to relate to them. And at that point I was
really so vulnerable, being recently, like, seroconverted, that, like, I didn't
want to deal with white dudes . . . basically . . . and white dudes hitting on me,
you know, in this moment of, like . . . where I felt, like, vulnerable sexually
or whatever. I'd rather deal with the straight dude at the HIV positive group,
you know, who was like, you know whatever. So I went to the straight support group. Which actually turned out to be more people of color, and a little
younger set, and a quarter of them were gay anyway.

This statement suggests that ICMNs should be central to any HIV intervention model for MLGBTQ2S populations. This individual, rather than choosing
a group of other gay men, chose a heterosexual group because of the painful
history associated with white colonialism, sexual abuse, and objectification.
However, while there are many concerns and potential problems with nonethnic-specific peer mentoring models, I do not want to understate the complexities also associated with the development of ICMNs. Some participants raised
significant concerns about the ongoing stereotypes and pan-Indian reductionist
approaches promoted by urban Indian organizations that lack tribal specificity:

I come in and everyone is all friendly and stuff, but sometimes they . . . I wish
there was more money for staff and there was no restrictions on blood quantum, or [questions about] are you enrolled? Or this or that. It's like, just if you
need help, we are here to help you. That would be lovely. Like, okay, that's
the restrictions I'm talking about, it's like, if you need . . . 'Cause that's what I
would do—if you need help, let me help you. 'Cause there was a lady crying
in the train station today, just this old woman sitting in the corner crying on
the ground. And I went and talked to her and I offered to buy her some cold
medicine or whatever she needed. And she was doing all right and says, "Will
you just talk to me?" So I sat for fifteen minutes and talked to her. She said
thank you! And I shook her hand and I said, "I hope you feel better." But she
goes, "That helped." Even that little tiny bit, even though I didn't do anything,
I just talked to her. But to offer no restrictions, you don't have to give me any
money, whatever you need please let me help you. That would be nice . . . in a
perfect world.

Internalizing the ideologies of colonizing nations continues to deeply impact
the delivery of health care services in Indigenous communities, as the previous
quote demonstrates. If Native-specific organizations are to effectively reduce

HIV/AIDS risk, they must shift away from colonial policies and practices that focus on blood quantum and enrollment restrictions, and toward high-quality services based on a shared sense of community, urban cultural affinities, and participation. Cultural competence as discussed thus far is a foundational component of building an urban Indian kinship network of support, but without a high standard of service delivery, cultural competence may not be enough to prevent MLGBTQ2S people from choosing nonethnic-specific efficiency over ethnic-specific cultural competence.

> I think, like, some basic competence would help, first of all. Sometimes I go into a clinic or something, and there might be staff, they might be ethnically, culturally competent. But when you wanna get something done, they have no clue of how to treat people. Like, you know, it takes them forever to do something for you that should—that they should just know how to do what needs to be done. So, like, there's this baseline of confidence, you know, that should exist. Um . . . and they should be efficient. That's why I'd rather go to somebody who is not culturally competent who is gonna be efficient with my care. Then on top of that, it's icing on the cake if they have some competence. . . . You know, 'cause I go to Kaiser and my physician is really competent. My nurse calls back when I call her, she picks up the phone, she answers me. She tries to do the best that she can, and I feel that. And that's what gives me confidence, you know, in the services. Yeah. And then like, secondly, it's like, um . . . yeah, it would be nice to like have, you know, folks who were like gay in the end. At all levels of the staff, not just the frontline staff. 'Cause often you go to, like, a Native organization and the frontline staff is like maybe Indian, and the middle management are, like, white or Asian, and then the very top are, like you know, these Indian moguls. Who, like, lord it over everybody else and use the middle management to, like, control everybody else. I think that's actually the case here in San Francisco at the health center, and stuff like that. And I think that's a problem. Um . . . I think you need to have, like, Indian people in every single area of the organization straight up.

While this participant raises important points about the significance of having culturally competent and efficient services that include gay and Native staff at all levels of Native organizations, it is a struggle for American Indian organizations and health agencies to recruit an entirely Native staff, due to the small overall size of the population and to the shortage of Natives in the field of medicine in general and of HIV/AIDS treatment in particular. This is not to suggest that Native organizations should not reassess the institutional culture and structure of their facilities, but it is equally important to point out that many ethnic-specific organizations lack the external funding to build stronger capacity and are often in competition with other organizations for grants that will allow them to produce more efficient programs that include more Native and MLGBTQ2S staff.

Constructing tribally specific ICMNs remains difficult in urban Indian communities because it is a challenge to match those who need mentoring with mentors from the same tribes. One possible solution to this dilemma is the co-construction and codevelopment of a shared definition of TUICKS among MLGBTQ2S mentors and mentees. Sharing the responsibility for cocreating TUICKS addresses at least two of the major concerns of MLGBTQ2S American Indians. First, the conflation of Indian or pan-Indian traditions with those of tribally specific nations can finally be taken off the table as a concern if we make space for at least two forms of regional/culturally specific traditional knowledge: urban and tribal. Second, a cocreation process for TUICKS can provide the space to deconstruct tribal-specific hegemony in the construction of pan-Indian narratives of "authenticity." In the Bay Area, tribes such as the Lakota and Cherokee are often cited by other Natives as dominant in the construction of Native cultural practices and representations visible to non-Natives as well as other Indigenous people. An exchange between two focus group participants highlights these tensions and can be read as a call for new narratives and approaches to defining urban Indian identity.

No, I think it's good to have a mix of people. But when I go back to Oklahoma and to Cherokee Services . . . our nation is different from other Indian nations, so you can't lump all American Indians in the same group. People in Oklahoma who have a longer history of assimilation and contact with whites are more assimilated to White culture, even blood quantum-wise. My tribe is, there are very few full-bloods left. And most everybody is mixed race, that's just the way it is. Whereas if you go to, like, Navajo land, there's tons of full-bloods. So, to try to just lump Navajos and Cherokees, just because we are both Native American Indians, it's like, you're gonna be looking for different things. The Navajos are gonna expect different things than the Cherokee. Um . . . so . . . I don't know how to solve that. Yeah, I think that would be a conundrum.

And actually, you bring up an excellent point—it's kind of ethnic domination, you know . . . And I think I said "honoring and respecting," and if I didn't, one of the things I meant is honoring and respecting. And it's the assumptions that you're Dine or Lakota, and these are the ways and . . . That's part of the urban dynamic, especially within San Francisco and . . . Red Power, Pan-Indianism, and those other ism-schisms, but . . . as a community, um . . . sometimes we forget to honor and embrace our differences. We'd much rather focus in on, um . . . what our ethereal commonalities are, and it's actually that repracticing of racism. And just this blank stereotype of what it is, and rather than dealing with the human being. 'Cause that's what it's really about, is embracing the human being. And if there are those commonalities of, our cultural commonalities, then, you know, great! That's all the gravy. But human services . . . [those are] two key words.

Both participants speak to the ill effects of the over-homogenization of Indigenous peoples and tribal nations into one generic "Indian" category, and of missing the unique and varied histories of colonialism among different American Indian tribal nations. There is also an indictment here of the ways that hegemony takes form in urban Indian environments, where the influence, cultural practices, and histories of larger tribes such as the Lakota, Cherokee, and Dine can sometimes overshadow those of other Native groups. In the Bay Area, for example, California Indians are often overshadowed by nations from other regions of the country. These monolithic representations of "the" Native as always already Lakota or Cherokee, for example, can also lead to cultural appropriation of Lakota and Cherokee language and traditions by urban Indians who lack a tribally specific connection to their own nations. Therefore, it is urgent that, as we discuss and trace a dual or multinational tradition among urban Indians, we accept the ability of Natives to be culturally fluent both in respect to their own tribes and in regards to their own traditional urban Indian communities where they, their parents, and grandparents may have grown up and participated in the development of TUICKS.

In this way, MLGBTQ2S Natives can continue to demonstrate a deep commitment to the decolonization of gender, sexuality, and mixed-race identity as necessary components to reducing HIV risk, while building intergenerational networks of support, peer mentoring, and cultural leadership that will strengthen the urban Indian community in the San Francisco Bay Area.

INTERGENERATIONAL HEALING
AND CULTURAL LEADERSHIP

MLGBTQ2S elders are a difficult population to define and identify because not everyone becomes an elder simply because they reach a certain age. In the context of the San Francisco Bay Area urban Indian community, I define an elder as someone who has been identified by the community as an elder as a result of their participation, leadership, and cultural knowledge of Native history in the region over an extended period of time from the 1970s onward. One participant's thinking about becoming such an elder reflect a sentiment I often hear within the Two-Spirit and LGBTQ American Indian community in the Bay Area:

> Well, when I first came out here [to San Francisco], there were so many different Indian people from so many different tribes, you know. And we were just so young and wide-eyed. . . . Many of us had been through boarding schools and then relocation. And so um, many of us, you know, we had strong ties to our tribes and our traditions and we brought that traditional knowledge with us to the Bay Area. There were gay American Indians at Alcatraz and many of us joined in the Red Power movement to make our voices and stories more, like, visible, you know. We had a strategy to go to the media to be sure people saw us, you know, at like Pride parades and powwows and what not. And today a lot of that generation that started groups like Gay American Indians, we're getting older and dying off, and there is, like, a gap or disconnect sometimes that I worry about in terms of that leadership and tight community that I felt we had. But I also see some hope, you know, with these young people in BAAITS and others that organize the Two-Spirit powwows and other wellness types of things. We need to—well I would like to . . . um, before it's too late, see more intergenerational spaces to ensure that gay Indians and lesbians, and Two-Spirits don't stop the momentum that we built up over so many years. It's like I worry sometimes and I feel blessed that I learned all those ceremonies and ways of my tribe and at the same time, when I came here we made these new traditions. We struggled a lot and with the AIDS epidemic, I saw a lot of those young Indian activists die before their time, and I wish they could see how things have—how things are kind of changing. But I know we have to get together more the elders and new generation and get past any drama created by non-Indians, and sometimes to be honest that we create ourselves, so we can live with more dignity and more honor, you know what

I mean? We need to have leaders so we don't lose everything we've gained through the years. I try to do my part and I'll talk to any young person interested in this Indian community and if I can help them learn about their own tribe, I've done that too.

As this elder attests—and as I've been told by elders, young people, educators, and activists—intergenerational healing can happen if the community can deal with the divisions and internal struggles that exist as a result of adopting non-Native ideologies of tradition, race, gender, and sexuality. In expressing his concern about the future leadership of the community and the need to protect some of the important strides that have been made by previous and contemporary ethnic- and LGBTQ-specific organizations, this elder also suggests that preserving urban traditions alongside tribally specific traditions is possible if there is a space for this type of dialogue. As this book has suggested, questions of "authenticity" around what constitutes tradition create deeply embedded resentments and hostilities in some urban Indian communities (Fixico 2000). Considering these debates about authenticity helps to explain why the term Two-Spirit gives some Natives pause when, it is assumed, outsiders are using the term in inappropriate ways. Because such questions affect the MLGBTQ2S population, I want to open up a dialogue among scholars, activists, and community members about regionally specific understandings of the term Two-Spirit and about how different communities come to understand and identify with the concept and practice. In other words, I want to propose that the Bay Area Two-Spirit community can serve as a case study here for the development and understanding of other urban Indian, Two-Spirit communities across the United States. As scholars study the urbanization of Native people, they will find unique cultural systems that have been developed by urban Indian groups, organizations, and families in virtually every major city where Native people came as a result of relocation. These studies will go along way in explicating the histories, identities, and future directions that must be taken to address, on a case-by-case basis, the health concerns not just of MLGBTQ2S people, but of all American Indians living in urban areas, by identifying the specific TUICKS of each region and city.

Two-Spirit, as discussed in earlier chapters, is a contested term that is not used here to represent all tribes or urban Indian communities. Achieving urban Two-Spirit return requires that Two-Spirit identities and communities be understood as always constructed within genealogies of history, place, and culture. I have argued that Two-Spirit sensibilities, while diverse, do share common narratives that attempt to move away from Western colonial constructions of gender and sexuality as always already fixed or binary. In the San Francisco Bay Area, Two-Spirit community members and Two-Spirit organizations are creating their own unique and specific traditional practices that contribute to the formation of this region's TUICKS. It is within this context that a return to noncolonial, Indigenous worldviews is taking place. While there are many different tribal nations represented in this Indigenous region of the country, it is precisely this heterogeneity that has become a central aspect of tradition for the generations of Native peoples who have relocated to the Bay Area over the past six decades, as well as among those California Natives whose ancestors have lived here for millennia. In order to return to a noncolonial or decolonial practice of gender, sexual, and ethnic diversity, urban MLGBTQ2S populations must enter into critical dialogues with one another about the ongoing legacies and impacts of intergenerational trauma.

These cross and intergenerational dialogues, when centered on healing, can open up the conditions and possibilities for decolonization, through active and critical engagement of kinship networks that work to heal the mistrust, pain, and trauma associated with Two-Spirit dissolution and PTIS. If MLGBTQ2S people are to reduce their risk for HIV infection, they must have a cultural structure in place to buffer the ongoing impact of the IBPN risk factors. During participant and community discussions during the course of my research collaboration with NAAP, at least one tangible intervention model rose to the surface as a possible means not simply to reduce HIV risk, but also to strengthen community cohesion and self-determination among MLBGTQ2S American Indians in the San Francisco Bay Area.

The intergenerational healing and cultural leadership (IHCL) intervention model, presented below, initially was a proposal for the implementation of a two-year, multisite intervention that would provide the empirical data necessary to assess MLGBTQ2S service needs regarding ethnic specific, community-based networks of support (see Table 8.1). The intervention design also sought to restore and increase the cultural networks of support that Two-Spirit people both provide and benefit from within American Indian communities. As the research unfolded, it became clear that the intervention should begin as a one-site intervention in the San Francisco Bay Area, in order to understand the regionally specific context of Two-Spirit practices in this area, without assuming a priori knowledge of the other originally proposed additional sites in Los Angeles and Seattle. The current model proposes a one-site intervention in partnership with the NAHC offices in San Francisco and Oakland, in collaboration with members of the BAAITS organization. The goal of the intervention is to produce effective urban Indian kinship networks of support and healing that link different generations of mixed-blood American Indians. If successful, this model will provide the community with another method to combat intergenerational trauma and Two-Spirit cultural dissolution while simultaneously reducing HIV risk among MLGBTQ2S people.

TABLE 8.1. Intergenerational Healing and Cultural Leadership Model

Research design	Conduct an intervention at Native American health centers in San Francisco and Oakland
Year One	
Phase 1	Recruit twenty-five elders (over 45 years of age) to partner with youth
Phase 2	Conduct training and focus group sessions for elders group, to discuss cultural retention, Two-Spirit leadership, and intergenerational trauma
Phase 3	Recruit twenty-five mixed-race Native youth (between 18 and 45 years of age)
Phase 4	Conduct training and focus group sessions with youth group, to discuss cultural retention, Two-Spirit leadership, and intergenerational trauma
Year Two	
Phase 5	Hold cultural summit and ceremony of return and homecoming, to welcome Two-Spirits back into community as cultural leaders
Phase 6	Hold talking circles and one-on-one mentoring sessions to develop community participation plans, which will be assessed at six-month and twelve-month periods, during gathering of participants and community based-organizations
Phase 7	Present actions taken by youth to become more involved in the Native community as cultural leaders, including impact statement from each participant about how the experience affected him or her personally in terms of behavior, stress, and wellness. Develop a stress and wellness rubric to assess the effectiveness of the model on participants. Publish data and rubrics in peer-review journals. Utilize any additional funding to focus on a national intervention.

Months after completing the research for this book, I took time to reflect on the importance of the data that was collected and how the specific stories of each participant contributed to similar themes around colonial trauma, kinship, healing, and intergenerational leadership. What became clear to me the more I reflected was that the most important aspect of this model is the premise that it be codeveloped by and from MLGBTQ2S perspectives and experiences. This is why I propose an intervention model that is a collaboration between Bay Area American Indian Two-Spirits and the Native American Health Center, so that as many MLGBTQ2S people as possible can participate in the design and implementation. It is my hope that this intergenerational healing and leadership model will encourage the further development of both community-based and scholarly understandings of the significance of TUICKS in dismantling the colonial traumas that continue to place Indigenous peoples at risk for HIV infection.

As many Indigenous scholars have noted, responsibility for Indigenous knowledge creation, education, and self-determination in research must be placed in the hands of the community members most directly impacted by colonization (Smith 1999, Mihesuah and Cavendar-Wilson 2004, Wilson and Yellow Bird 2005, Abu-Saad and Champagne 2006, Wilson 2009). Therefore, as I reflected further I began to realize that even the very proposal of this IHCL model would have to be vetted and reassessed by members of San Francisco's Two-Spirit community.

The first year of the two-year intervention involves the recruitment of twenty-five elders (ideally elders will be forty-five years of age and older, but the final definition of an elder will be determined by members of the advisory board at NAHC, which includes community members, academics, and medical professionals, and by BAAITS members. Once the elders are recruited, a focus group session and training codesigned by elder participants, NAHC staff, and BAAITS members will allow mentors to discuss and identify key themes and needs related to cultural retention, leadership cultivation, and the reduction of intergenerational trauma. One challenge with such an intervention is identifying and recruiting participants: in conversations with local tribal leaders, the desire for mentors is frequently raised, but often the sentiment is that while there is a strong desire for peer and intergenerational mentoring programs, there is a lack of available mentors. In addressing this potential recruitment challenge I propose casting a wide net to recruit as many participants as possible from a range of American Indian nations. In the San Francisco Bay Area, that would mean working not only with former members of Gay American

Indians, NAAP, and BAAITS, but also with local California tribal communities, reservations, and rancherias, all of which are often ignored in such efforts due to distance and insufficiently developed relationships. Many members of these communities, while firmly rooted in their own specific tribal traditions, also actively participate in the cultivation and development of TUICKS and would therefore make appropriate mentors, as well as mentees. The third and fourth phases of year one include the recruitment of twenty-five Native youth mentees (ideally under the age of forty-five, though the final definition of Native youth can be determined by the advisory board and members of the BAAITS organization) followed by a focus group session and training codesigned by youth participants BAAITS members and NAHC staff.

The second year of the IHCL intervention model is envisioned as beginning with a MLGBTQ2S cultural summit and ceremony of return and reconciliation, cocreated by participants, advisory board members, and agency staff to incorporate TUICKS unique to the San Francisco Bay Area Indian community. I envision the ceremony as a moment to reprioritize Indigenous epistemologies from both urban and tribal frameworks of cultural knowledge and community. Such a ceremony may offer an opportunity for MLGBTQ2S people to reconcile antagonistic experiences of internal and external rejection in the face of colonial haunting; microaggressions based on mixed-race identity, gender, and sexuality; as well as the ongoing influences of settler colonialism on Indigenous-determined group membership criteria.

During the second year, it is envisioned that youth and elders will come together to meet and conduct talking circles and one-on-one mentoring sessions. As with all mentoring programs, it's likely that there will be bidirectional mentoring and that many of the youth participants will also provide important knowledge to their mentors. As elder and youth participants begin the mentoring process, they will be asked to create and complete risk-behavior and stress-coping rubrics, to measure the ways that they currently deal with stress and with high-risk sexual and social behavior. Elder and youth participants will also be asked to identify potential goals for reducing stress and mitigating high-risk behavior in the context of collective and communal healing, as opposed to individual therapies and intervention approaches. To this end, youth and elders will collectively establish community participation action plans during the second year of the program, for assessment after six months. At the end of the second year of participation in the IHCL intervention model, all participants will report on the status of their community action plans during a summit meeting with all fifty participants. Youth will report on their progress in taking up cultural leadership positions within the community, and elders will discuss their efforts in supporting their mentees in implementing their community action plans. Each participant will also present an impact statement about how personal effects of the IHCL experience in terms of behavior, stress, and wellness will be measured according to the stress and wellness rubrics designed by participants.

The IHCL intervention seeks to create a model for American Indian healing among MLGBTQ2S individuals who are currently at risk for HIV/AIDS. If successful, this model can be used to bring new knowledge and practices to the fields of queer studies, public health, and Native American studies. As a cocreated, coowned model, the approach in and of itself, addresses many of the challenges identified throughout this book for MLGBTQ2S people. Decolonization is ultimately a question of obtaining and sharing the power to define one's experience, history, and identity with other members of the community without colonial influence. MLGBTQ2S American Indians, in cocreating this intervention, will obtain and share this power to name their own experiences, an important first step in healing and ending colonial haunting.

The IHCL intervention model also seeks to queer public health discourse by offering new ethnic-specific and culturally competent approaches to HIV/AIDS prevention from an inter- and transdisciplinary perspective. As MLGBTQ2S people move to the center from the most marginalized spaces in studies dealing with HIV/AIDS in Indigenous communities, more nuanced and pragmatic critical interrogations of anti-Indianism and public health disparities will emerge. The IHCL model is just one recommended step in a long process toward decolonization and cultural healing.

Intervention models in American Indian communities must consider two important concepts: communal healing and intergenerational love. In reflecting on my own life as a mixed-blood, American Indian man living with HIV/AIDS, I am conscious of the innumerable ways that people within the communities that I come from are often forced to live life in the shadows, as invisible people devoid of ethnic and cultural identities. The writing of this book from beginning to end has reminded me that wellness and healing from colonial trauma has to begin with self-determination. When I consider the stories of the MLGBTQ2S people who contributed to the collective narrative that is *Indian Blood*, I must acknowledge that the initial seeds of decolonization are being planted every day that we tell our stories.

In every instance that we as Indigenous people come together to collectively make our stories known, we are healing not only individually, but also as a community. It is in this process of telling our stories and achieving communal healing that we open up a process for articulating intergenerational love. More than five centuries of colonial haunting have led to many forms of trauma and nihilism in Native communities across the United States. Today, as I remember and share the stories and wisdom of those who contributed to *Indian Blood* as a diverse community of Two-Spirit people, I realize that the most effective intervention we have in reducing high-risk behavior and the spread of HIV is intergenerational love. Learning to love ourselves and those generations that came before and who will come after is so important for creating and maintaining mental, spiritual, and physical health.

Intergenerational love means that we have to forgive. We must forgive ourselves and we must forgive our ancestors. It also means we have to channel our anger and our experiences with trauma into action steps. And with every action that we take as individuals and as a community, the closer we come to returning to a sacred place, where healing silences the sounds of the haunting. We must silence the sounds of the haunting so that we may hear our ancestors speaking to us as they call out, "We love you. Our lifeblood sustains you. Take every step you can knowing that we walk with you toward healing, toward balance." And so in the end, each of us must remember that every step towards wellness, every step towards inclusivity, and every step towards holistic health in the face of colonial haunting and HIV will bring us that much closer to the day when the decolonization of gender, sexuality, and mixed-race identity categories leads to a truly sovereign, self-determined American Indian community.

NOTES

1   The concept of research as ceremony is articulated by Cree scholar Shawn Wilson in his 2009 book, *Research Is Ceremony: Indigenous Research Methods*. The term *research justice* was established by the DataCenter Research for Justice in Oakland. For more information, go to www.datacenter.org/.

2   In her 2008 essay "Conjugating Subjects in the Age of Multiculturalism," Nora Alarcon argues that identity and differences in identity allow people to express their subjectivity by constantly defining what it means to be a person "belonging" to a particular identity. In this book, I examine the ways that Two-Spirit, LGBT, and queer-identified mixed-race American Indians constantly renegotiate and define who they are by exposing the contradictions created by researchers who create strict and universal definitions to define group membership.

3   The Cass model, developed in 1970 by Vivienne Cass, created a model of "homosexual" identity development comprised of six stages that a gay or lesbian person goes through while exploring and understanding their own identity. The model has been critiqued for its binary treatment of sexual identity categories (lesbian, gay) and for its linear model of identity stages for people who identify as queer. The six stages, in order, are: identity confusion, identity comparison, identity tolerance, identity acceptance, identity pride, identity synthesis. While this model has some validity for non-Native people, it runs counter to many of the historical ways in which the ancestors of MLGBTQ2S people would have developed or come to understand their roles and responsibilities as they related to gender and sexuality. Though the Cass Model was one of the first theories to treat homosexuality as a "normal" expression of sexual orientation, it nevertheless creates a one-dimensional, Western European model for explaining "homosexual" identity development without taking into consideration variation in queer identity development across different cultural and ethnic groups.

4   Jacobs, Thomas, and Lang (1997) discuss the meanings of specific terms, including *nádleehé* among the Navajo, which refers to someone in a constant process of change, and *winkte* among the Siouan groups, used to describe people who took on dual or multiple gender roles. The authors note however, that "these terms do not refer to sexual behavior," but have to do with gender roles and responsibilities—although they also note that such gender role(s) did not preclude the possibility of same-sex relations.

2. TWO-SPIRIT CULTURAL DISSOLUTION

1   Two-Spirits in many, but not all tribal communities, are individuals who historically practiced gender balance between male and female genders. In some tribal societies, such as the Zuni (see Will Roscoe [1998], *Changing Ones: Third and Fourth Genders in Native North America*) Two-Spirits were not seen as homosexual, transgender, or gay, as they might be in a contemporary context. Instead, Two-Spirits were often religious and

ceremonial leaders who held a special place in tribal life because they represented a balance of gender identity and therefore were seen as special keepers of knowledge. Attacks
on the practices of Two-Spirits by European religious leaders during colonization caused
dissolution of the traditional roles they played in all facets of tribal life, from the religious
to the economic.

2   A soul wound is defined here as the loss of a spiritual and cultural connection to one's
      tribally specific worldview, as a result of centuries of historical trauma that leads to post-
      traumatic invasion syndrome (PTIS), which is then passed on to successive generations,
      causing not only a soul wound or loss of culture but the dissolution of traditional Two-
      Spirit protective factors. For more discussion of the soul wound concept, see Duran and
      Duran (1995).

3   The CDC (2010) elaborates on health disparities related to mixed-race American Indians
      and Alaskan Natives (AIAN), stating that "while the overall data reflects disparate rates
      of HIV/AIDS diagnoses, the larger contextual picture including multiplicity of Indigenous
      identity and experience may be obscured. Additionally, while the overall estimated num-
      ber and rate of AIDS diagnoses decreased between 2006 and 2009, it remained stable
      in AIAN communities (CDC 2009). In this same time period, HIV diagnoses increased
      despite an overall population decrease (CDC 2009) and this may be a better indicator
      of the HIV/AIDS risk in AIAN communities. Moreover, recent rates of infection among
      AIANs have increased more rapidly than in any other racial/ethnic group. In 1990, 223
      cases were reported and in 2001, 2537 cases: a 900% increase (Dennis 2009). Among
      individuals diagnosed with AIDS between 2001 and 2005, AIAN had shorter survival times
      than Whites, Asian and Pacific Islanders, multiple race, and Hispanics (CDC, 2009)."

3. HISTORICAL AND INTERGENERATIONAL TRAUMA AND RADICAL LOVE

1   Indian Health Services data from the late 1990s, as analyzed in Jones (2006), showed
      higher mortality rates among American Indians and Alaskan Natives compared with the
      general population for most leading causes of mortality: heart disease (1.2 times), acci-
      dents (2.8 times), diabetes (4.2 times), alcohol (7.7 times), suicide (1.9 times), and tuber-
      culosis (7.5 times). Only with cancer, the second leading cause of death, was American
      Indian mortality not greater than that of the general population. Furthermore, all of these
      disparities widened between 1995 and 1998.

4. GENDER AND RACIAL DISCRIMINATION
AGAINST MIXED-RACE AMERICAN INDIAN TWO-SPIRITS

1   In his 1999 book, *Disidentifications: Queers of Color and the Performance of Politics*,
      Muñoz looks at how those outside the racial and sexual mainstream negotiate majority
      culture, not by aligning themselves with or against exclusionary works but rather by
      transforming these works for their own cultural purposes.

2   *The Declining Significance of Race: Blacks and Changing American Institutions*, first pub-
      lished in 1980, was a contentious theorization by the prominent Harvard sociologist about
      the contours of class as more central in predicting the life chances of African Americans
      to gain social mobility in U.S. society. While heavily critiqued by many on the Left in
      academic and politics, Wilson's work catapulted him into the political arena in ways that
      few other sociologists have been able to attain. Throughout the 1990s, after his appoint-
      ment at Harvard University, Wilson was a key advisor to President Bill Clinton on issues

of poverty and inequality. I, along with many others, would mark the Clinton presidency as the "age of neoliberalism," when colorblind theories begin to eclipse clear linkages between ongoing inequality and poverty, and race and racism.

3   In *The Boundaries of Blackness: AIDS and the Breakdown of Black Politics*, Cathy Cohen argues that the individual members who sit on the furthest margins of Black communities often face "secondary marginalization" because their struggles and political interests are often not seen as the most salient topics to be addressed by the Black community. A similar process unfolds for American Indians, as I argue in chapter 1.

5. MIXED-RACE IDENTITY, COGNITIVE DISSONANCE, AND PUBLIC HEALTH

1   For more discussion of how mixed-blood and mixed-race Natives impact the urban public sphere and tribal politics, particularly through activism and supratribal and multitribal organizing, see Stephen Cornell, *The Return of the Native* (1990) and Joane Nagel, *American Indian Ethnic Renewal* (1997).

2   Jack Forbes has dealt extensively with the miscategorization of mixed-blood American Indians, especially those of mixed-African ancestry; see his 1993 work, *Africans and Native Americans*.

3   For further discussion of American Indian distrust of U.S. government agencies, and health and educational institutions, see United Nations (1977). According to that report, prepared in conjunction with Native American Solidarity Committee, 24 percent of Native women had been sterilized, 19 percent of whom were of child-bearing age (3). The report includes the following definition of genocide: "In the present Convention, genocide means any of the following acts committed with the intent to destroy, in whole or in part, a national, ethical, racial or religious group, as such: a) Killing members of the group; b) Causing serious bodily or mental harm to members of the group; c) Deliberately inflicting on the group conditions of life calculated to bring about its physical destruction in whole or in parts; d) Imposing measures intended to prevent births within a group; e) Forcibly transferring children of the group to another group" (1). Dillingham (1997), Deloria (1999), Duran and Duran (1995), and Pevar (1992) document American Indian mistrust of medical practices perpetrated by U.S. institutions that have a history of negligence, abuse, dishonesty, and genocide.

6. SEXUAL VIOLENCE AND TRANSFORMATIVE ANCESTOR SPIRITS

1   Information on VAWA actions in the Senate and the House of Representatives 2012 and 2013 was accessed through the YWCA website, www.ywca.org.

2   Data from the 2012 report can be obtained from the National Coalition of Anti-Violence Programs, www.avp.org/about-avp/coalitions-a-collaborations/82-national-coalition-of-anti-violence-programs.

3   Available at www2.ucsc.edu/rape-prevention/statistics.html.

4   Available at www2.ucsc.edu/rape-prevention/statistics.html.

5   In her 2000 book, *Methodology of the Oppressed*, Chela Sandoval offers her own theorization for how Third World feminists and feminists of color from marginalized groups can mobilize politically after forming their own ideologies, which often differ dramatically from those of mainstream white feminists. In this quote about her transgender identity, this participant is expressing a similar ideological approach, one that is both distinct from the mainstream and oppositional to Western constructions of normative gender identity.

7. STRESS COPING IN URBAN INDIAN KINSHIP NETWORKS

1   The concept of third generation return was first articulated by Marcus L. Hansen in his
    speech, "The Problem of the Third Generation Immigrant," to the Augustana Historical
    Society, in Rock Island, Illinois, in 1938.

2   Karl Mannheim, in his 1923 essay "The Problem of Generations," defines generational
    cohort groups as those who have lived through a similar set of historical events, which
    shaped a shared social consciousness. For example, Native youth who were the first gen-
    eration to be born in cities and not on reservations would constitute a generation, with
    a shared consciousness often tied to political events such as the Red Power movement
    and the rise of pan-Indianism. An NPR article, "Urban American Indians Rewrite Relo-
    cation's Legacy," documents the ways that the generation of children who came of age
    during relocation have been able to return to their tribes and support new programs that
    address intergenerational and historical trauma. Many of the children or grandchildren of
    those who were relocated are becoming more involved with their tribes, after completing
    degrees or after years of working in cities on issues related to Native displacement. For
    more discussion, see Hilliard 2012.

3   According to the Canadian AIDS Society, stress among Aboriginal women has been
    directly linked to increased drug and alcohol use as well as an increase in risk for contrac-
    tion of the HIV virus. Karina Walters and Jane Simoni, in their coauthored 2002 article,
    "Re-conceptualizing Native Women's Health: An 'Indigenist' Stress-Coping Model," argue
    that "the effect of life stressors (e.g., historical trauma) on health is moderated by cultural
    factors such as identity attitudes that function as buffers, strengthening psychological and
    emotional health and mitigating the effects of stressors."

4   Cultural influences on HIV risk have been documented by several scholars and the issue
    of finding appropriate tools to address cultural competence in HIV prevention was docu-
    mented by Julie Solomon, Jacqueline Berman, and Josefina Card in their 2007 book, *Tools
    for Building Culturally Competent HIV Prevention Programs.*

BIBLIOGRAPHY

Abu-Saad, Ismael, and Duane Champagne. 2006. *Indigenous Education and Empowerment: International Perspectives*. Lanham, MD: AltaMira Press.

Adams, Heather, and Layli Phillips. 2009. "Ethnic-Related Variations from the Cass Model of Homosexual Identity Formation: The Experiences of Two-Spirit, Lesbian, and Gay Native Americans." *Journal of Homosexuality* 56 (7): 959–76.

Alarcon, Norma. 2008. "Conjugating Subjects in the Age of Multiculturalism." In *Mapping Multiculturalism*, edited by Avery Gordon and Christopher Newfield, 127–48. Minneapolis: University of Minnesota Press.

Alfred, Taiaiake. 2009. *Peace, Power, and Righteousness: An Indigenous Manifesto*. Oxford: Oxford University Press.

Applegate Krouse, Susan. 1999. "Kinship and Identity: Mixed Bloods in Urban Indian Communities." *American Indian Culture and Research Journal* 23 (2): 73–89.

Aspin, Clive. 2011. "Exploring Takatapui Identity within the Maori Community: Implications for Health and Well-Being." In *Queer Indigenous Studies: Critical Interventions in Theory, Politics, and Literature,* edited by Qwo-Li Driskill, Chris Finley, Brian Joseph Gilley, and Scott Lauria Morgensen, 113–22. Tucson: University of Arizona Press.

Atkinson, Donald. 1979. *Counseling American Minorities: A Cross-Cultural Perspective*. Dubuque, Iowa: Brown.

Bandura, Albert. 1986. *Social Foundations of Thought and Action*. Englewood Cliffs, NJ: Prentice-Hall.

Banton, Michael. 1970. "The Concept of Racism." In *Race and Racialism*, edited by Sami Zubaida, 17–34. London: Tavistock.

Barker, Joanne. 2012. *Native Acts: Law, Recognition, and Cultural Authenticity*. Durham, NC: Duke University Press.

Barker, Joanne, ed. 2005. *Sovereignty Matters: Locations of Contestation and Possibility in Indigenous Struggles for Self-Determination*. Lincoln: University of Nebraska Press.

Blu, Karen. 2001 (1980). *The Lumbee Problem: The Making of an American Indian People*. Lincoln: University of Nebraska Press.

Bonilla-Silva, Eduardo. 1997. "Rethinking Racism: Toward a Structural Interpretation." *American Sociological Review* 62 (3): 465–80.

Browne, Angela, and David Finkelhor. 1986. "Impact of Child Sexual Abuse: A Review of the Research." *Psychological Bulletin* 99 (1): 66–77.

Buchwald, Dedra, Sue Tomita, and Spero Manson. 2000. "Physical Abuse of Urban Native Americans." *Journal of General Internal Medicine* 15 (8): 562–64.

Bureau of Indian Affairs, Office of Federal Acknowledgement. 2013. "Criteria to Establish Federal Recognition." www.bia.gov/WhoWeAre/AS-IA/OFA/. Accessed October 18, 2013.

Butler, Judith. 1993. *Gender Trouble: Feminism and the Subversion of Identity*. New York: Routledge.

Byrd, Jodi. 2011. *The Transit of Empire: Indigenous Critiques of Colonialism*. Minneapolis: University of Minnesota Press.

Canadian AIDS Society. 2012. "Injection Drug Use and HIV/AIDS." www.cdnaids.ca/. Accessed November 11, 2013.

Cass, Vivian. 1979. "Homosexual Identity Formation: A Theoretical Model." *Journal of Homosexuality* 4 (3): 219–35.

Centers for Disease Control. 2010. "American Indians and Alaska Native Populations." www.cdc. gov/minorityhealth/populations/REMP/aian.html. Accessed October 14, 2013.

Cheng, Patrick. 2011. *Radical Love: Introduction to Queer Theology.* New York: Seabury Books.

Choi, Yoonsun, Tracy Harachi, Mary Gillmore, and Richard Catalano. 2006. "Are Multiracial Adolescents at Greater Risk? Comparisons of Rates, Patterns and Correlates of Substance Use and Violence Between Monoracial and Multiracial Adolescents." *American Journal of Orthopsychiatry* 76 (1): 86–97.

Ciesla, Jeffrey, and John Roberts. 2001. "Meta-analysis of the Relationship between HIV Infection and Risk for Depressive Disorders." *American Journal of Psychiatry* 158 (5): 725–30.

Clements, Kristine, Rani Marx, Robert Guzman, S. Ikeda, and Mitchell Katz. 1998. "Prevalence of HIV Infection in Transgendered Individuals in San Francisco." Poster session presented at the Twelfth International Conference on AIDS, Geneva.

Cobb, Amanda. 2005. "Understanding Tribal Sovereignty: Definitions, Conceptualizations, and Interpretations." *American Studies* 46 (3/4): 115–32.

Cohen, Cathy. 1999. *The Boundaries of Blackness: AIDS and the Breakdown of Black Politics.* Chicago: University of Chicago Press.

Colorado, Pam. 1988. "Bridging Native and Western Science." *Convergence* 21 (2/3):. 49–69.

Connerton, Paul. 1989. *How Societies Remember.* Cambridge: Cambridge University Press.

Cook-Lynn, Elizabeth. 1996. "American Indian Intellectualism and the New Indian Story." *American Indian Quarterly* 20 (1): 57–76.

Cornell, Stephen. 1990. *The Return of the Native: American Indian Political Resurgence.* Oxford: Oxford University Press.

Cross, William. 1995. "The Psychology of Nigrescence: Revisiting the Cross Model." In *Handbook of Multicultural Counseling,* edited by Joseph Ponterotto, Manuel Casas, Lisa Suzuki, and Charlene Alexander, 93–122. Thousand Oaks, CA: Sage.

Cunningham, Jennifer. "Is Reverse Racism Real: An Interview with Eduardo Bonilla Silva." *The Grio.* http://thegrio.com/2010/08/18/is-reverse-racism-real/. Accessed October 18, 2013.

Dacosta, Kim. 2007. *Making Multiracials: State, Family, and Market in the Redrawing of the Color Line.* Stanford: Stanford University Press.

Daniel, G. Reginald. 2001. *More Than Black? Multiracial Identity and the New Racial Order.* Philadelphia: Temple University Press.

Darwin, Charles. 1859. *The Origin of Species.* London: John Murray Publishing.

———. 1871. "On the Races of Men . . . the Effects of Crossing." In *Mixed Race Studies: A Reader,* edited by Jayne Ifekwunigwe, 47–50. London: Routledge.

Davenport, Charles. 1929. *Race Crossing in Jamaica.* New York: Negro University Press.

de Count Gobineau, Joseph Arthur. 1853. "Recapitulation: The Respective Characteristics of the Three Great Races; The Superiority of the White Type, and within this Type, of the Aryan Family." In *Mixed Race Studies: A Reader,* edited by Jayne Ifekwunigwe, 208–11. London: Routledge.

Deloria, Vine, Jr. 1970. *We Talk, You Listen: New Tribes, New Turf.* New York: Macmillan.

———. 1999. *Tribes, Treaties, and Constitutional Tribulations.* Austin: University of Texas Press.

Deloria, Vine, Jr., and Clifford M. Lytle. 1984. *The Nations Within: The Past and Future of American Indian Sovereignty.* Austin: University of Texas Press.

Denetdale, Jennifer Nez. 2008. "Carving Navajo National Boundaries: Patriotism, Tradition, and the Diné Marriage Act of 2005." *American Indian Quarterly* 60 (2): 280–94.

Diaz, Rafael. 1997. *Latino Gay Men and HIV: Culture, Sexuality.* New York: Routledge.

Diaz, Rafael, and Ayala, George. 2011. *Social Discrimination and Health: The Case of Latino Gay Men and HIV Risk.* New York: National Gay and Lesbian Task Force.

Dillingham, Brint. 1977. "American Indian Women and the IHS Sterilization Practices." *American Indian Journal of the Institute for the Development of Indian Law* 3: 27–28.

Ditewig-Morris, Kate, Hannabah Blue, and Jamie Folsom. 2011. "Addressing Historical Trauma: The Struggle of Native American Women against HIV/AIDS." U.S. National Native American AIDS Prevention Center. www.thebody.com/content/art61027.html. Accessed October 14, 2013.

Dominguez, Virginia. 1993. *White by Definition: Social Classification in Creole Louisiana.* New Brunswick, NJ: Rutgers University Press.

Driskill, Qwo-Li. 2008. "Shaking Our Shells: Cherokee Two-Spirits Rebalancing the World." In *Beyond Masculinity: Essays by Queer Men on Gender and Politics,* edited by Trevor Hoppe, n.p. www.beyondmasculinity.com/articles/.

Driskill, Qwo-Li, Chris Finley, Brian Giley, and Scott Morgensen. 2011. *Queer Indigenous Studies: Critical Interventions in Theory, Politics, and Literature.* Tucson: University of Arizona Press.

Duran, Bonnie, and Duran, Eduardo. 1995. *Native American Postcolonial Psychology.* Albany: SUNY Press.

Fergusson, David L., John Horwood, Elizabeth M. Ridder, and Annette L. Beautrais. 2005. "Sexual Orientation and Mental Health in a Birth Cohort of Young Adults." *Psychological Medicine* 35 (7): 97–81.

Finley, Chris. 2011. "Decolonizing the Queer Body (and Recovering the Native Bull-Dyke): Bringing 'Sexy Back' and Out of Native Studies' Closet." In *Queer Indigenous Studies: Critical Interventions in Theory, Politics, and Literature,* edited by Qwo-Li Driskill, Chris Finley, Brian Giley, and Scott Morgensen, 31–42. Tucson: University of Arizona Press.

Fisher, Jeffrey and William Fisher. 1992. "Changing AIDS-Risk Behavior." *Psychology Bulletin* 111 (3): 455–74.

Fixico, Donald. 2000. *The Urban Indian Experience in America.* Albuquerque: University of New Mexico Press.

Forbes, Jack. 1993. *Africans and Native Americans: The Language of Race and the Evolution of Red-Black Peoples.* Champaign: University of Illinois Press.

Foucault, Michel. 1972. *Power/Knowledge: Selected Interviews and Other Writings, 1972–1977,* edited by Colin Gordon. New York: Pantheon Books.

Futures without Violence. Violence against Women Fact Sheet. www.futureswithoutviolence.org/userfiles/file/Violence%20Against%20AI%20AN%20Women%20Fact%20Sheet.pdf. Accessed November 11, 2013.

Galton, Francis. 1869. *Hereditary Genius.* London: Macmillan and Company.

Garroutte, Eva. 2002. *Real Indians: Identity and the Survival of Native America.* Los Angeles: University of California Press.

Giley, Brian. 2006. *Becoming Two-Spirit: Gay Identity and Social Acceptance in Indian Country.* Lincoln: University of Nebraska Press.

Goeman, Mishuana. 2013. *Mark My Words: Native Women Mapping Our Nations.* Minneapolis: University of Minnesota Press.

Gomez-Barris, Macarena. 2008. *Where Memory Dwells: Culture and State Violence in Chile.* Berkeley: University of California Press.

Gordon, Avery. 2008. *Ghostly Matters: Haunting and the Sociological Imagination.* Minneapolis: University of Minnesota Press.

Greenwood, Gregory, Michael Relf, Bu Huang, Lance Pollack, Jesse Canchola, and Joesph Catania. 2002. "Battering Victimization among a Probability-Based Sample of Men Who Have Sex with Men." *American Journal of Public Health* 92 (12): 1964–69.

Hansen, Marcus L. 1938. "The Problem of the Third Generation Immigrant." Paper presented at the Augustana Historical Society, Rock Island, Illinois. MSS 203, Augustana Historical Society records, Special Collections, Augustana College.

Hays, Robert, Gregory Rebchook, and Susan Kegeles. 2003. "The Mpowerment Project: Commu-
nity-Building with Young Gay and Bisexual Men to Prevent HIV1." *American Journal of Community Psychology* 31 (3–4): 301–12.

Helms, Janel. 1995. "An Update of Helms's White and People of Color Racial Identity Development
Models." In *Handbook of Multicultural Counseling*, edited by Joseph Ponterotto, Manuel Casas,
Lisa Suzuki, and Charlene Alexander, 181–98. Thousand Oaks, CA: Sage.

Hilliard, Gloria. 2012. "Urban American Indians Rewrite Relocations Legacy." www.npr.
org/2012/01/07/143800287/urban-american-indians-rewrite-relocations-legacy. Accessed
November 11, 2013.

Hixson, Walter L. 2013. *American Settler Colonialism: A History.* New York: Palgrave Macmillan.

Hotakainen, Rob. 2013. "Among Indian Tribes, a Division over Gay Marriage." *Washington Post,*
May 13, 2013.

Ifekwunigwe, Jayne. 2004. *Mixed Race Studies: A Reader.* New York: Routledge.

Incite! 2009. *The Revolution Will Not Be Funded: Beyond the Non-Profit Industrial Complex.* Cambridge: South End Press.

Jacobs, Sue-Ellen, Wesley Thomas, and Sabine Lang. 1997. *Two-Spirit People: Native American Gender Identity, Sexuality, and Spirituality.* Urbana: University of Illinois Press.

Johnson, Kevin. 2003. *Mixed-Race Americans and the Law: A Reader.* New York: New York University Press.

Jolivette, Andrew J. 2007. *Louisiana Creoles: Cultural Recovery and Mixed Race Native American
Identity.* Lanham, MD: Lexington Books.

———. 2012. "Barack Obama and the Rise to Power: Emmett Till Revisited." In *Obama and the
Biracial Factor: The Battle for a New American Majority*, edited by Andrew J. Jolivette. Bristol,
UK: Policy Press.

———. 2015. "Research Justice: Radical Love as a Strategy for Social Transformation." In *Research
Justice: Methodologies for Social Change*, edited by Andrew J. Jolivette. Bristol, UK: Policy Press.

Jones, David. 2006. "The Persistence of American Indian Health Disparities." *American Journal of
Public Health* 96 (12): 2122–34.

Kelly, J. A., D. A. Murphy, K. J. Sikkema, T. L. McAuliffe, R. A. Roffman, L. J. Solomon, R. A. Winett.
1997. "Randomised, Controlled, Community-Level HIV-Prevention Intervention for Sexual-
Risk Behaviour among Homosexual Men in US Cities." *Lancet* 350 (9090): 1500–5.

Kitano, Harry, Wai-Tsang Yeung, Lynn Chai, and Herbert Hatanaka. 1984. "Asian American Interracial Marriage." *Journal of Marriage and Family* 46 (1): 179–90.

Klopotek, Brian. 2011. *Recognition Odysseys: Indigeneity, Race, and Federal Tribal Recognition Policy
in Three Louisiana Indian Communities.* Durham, NC: Duke University Press.

———. 2012. "Dangerous Decolonizing: Indians and Blacks and the Legacy of Jim Crow." In *Decolonizing Native Histories: Collaboration, Knowledge, and Language in the Americas*, edited by
Florencia E. Mallon, 178–94. Durham, NC: Duke University Press.

Knox, Robert. 1850. "Do Races Ever Amalgamate?" In *Mixed Race Studies: A Reader*, edited by Jayne
Ifekwunigwe, 37–38. London: Routledge.

Latkin, Carl, Susan Sherman, and Amy Knowlton. 2003. "HIV Prevention among Drug Users: Out-
come of a Network-Oriented Peer Outreach Intervention." *Health Psychology* 22 (4): 332–39.

Lee, Sharon, and Barry Edmonston. 2005. "New Marriages, New Families: U.S. Racial and Hispanic
Intermarriage." *Population Bulletin* 60 (2): 3–36.

Lobo, Susan, and Kurt Peters. 2001. *American Indians and the Urban Experience.* Lanham, MD:
AltaMira Press.

Lyons, Scott Richard. 2000. "Rhetorical Sovereignty: What Do American Indians Want from Writing?" *College Composition and Communication* 51 (3): 447–68.

Mannheim, Karl. 1923. "The Problem of Generations." In *Essays on the Sociology of Knowledge*. London: RKP.

Martin, James I., Jo G. Pryce, and James D. Leeper. 2005. "Avoidance Coping and HIV Risk Behavior among Gay Men." *Health Social Work* 30 (3): 193–201.

Mellers, Barbara, Alan Schwartz, Katty Ho, and Ilana Ritov. 1997. "Decision Affect Theory: Emotional Reactions to Outcomes of Risky Options." *Psychological Science* 8 (6): 423–29.

Mihesuah, Devon, and Angela Cavendar-Wilson. 2004. *Indigenizing the Academy: Transforming Scholarship and Empowering Communities*. Lincoln: University of Nebraska Press.

Miles, Robert. 1989. *Racism after "Race Relations."* London: Routledge.

———. 1993. "The Articulation of Racism and Nationalism: Reflections on European History." In *Racism and Migration in Western Europe*, edited by John Wrench and John Solomos, 35–52. Oxford: Berg Publishers.

Miles, Tiya. 2006. *The Ties that Bind: The Story of an Afro-Cherokee Family in Slavery and Freedom*. Berkeley: University of California Press.

Morgensen, Scott. 2011. *Spaces between Us: Queer Settler Colonialism and Indigenous Decolonization*. Minneapolis: University of Minnesota Press.

Muñoz, José E. 1999. *Disidentifications: Queers of Color and the Performance of Politics*. Minneapolis: University of Minnesota Press.

Nagel, Joane. 1997. *American Indian Ethnic Renewal: Red Power and the Resurgence of Identity and Culture*. Oxford: Oxford University Press.

National Alliance of State and Territorial AIDS Directors. 2008. "Technical Assistance Report: Activities to Address HIV/AIDS in Native American Communities." www.ncminorityhealth.org/data/documents/NativeAmericanHIVReport.pdf. Accessed October 14, 2013.

National Coalition of Anti-Violence Programs. "2012 Report on Lesbian, Gay, Bisexual, Transgender, Queer, and HIV-Affected Intimate Partner Violence." www.avp.org/resources/avp-resources/273. Accessed November 10, 2013.

National Gay and Lesbian Task Force. 2012. "Injustice at Every Turn: A Look at American Indian and Alaskan Native Respondents in the National Transgender Discrimination Survey." www.thetaskforce.org/injustice-every-turn-look-american-indian-alaskan-native-respondents-national-transgender-discrimination-survey/. Accessed October 16, 2013.

Native American AIDS Project. 2012. "NAAP's Announcement." December 15, 2012. http://naap-ca.org (site discontinued).

Nott, Josiah Clark, and George Robins Gliddon. 1854. "Hybridity of Animals, Viewed in Connection with the Natural History of Mankind." In *Mixed Race Studies: A Reader*, edited by Jayne Ifekwunigwe, 42–46. London: Routledge.

Odell-Korgen, Kathleen. 2010. *Multiracial Americans and Social Class*. New York: Routledge.

Paul, Jay, Joseph Catania, Lance Pollack, and Ronald Stall. 2001. "Understanding Childhood Sexual Abuse as a Predictor of Sexual Risk-Taking among Men who have Sex with Men: The Urban Men's Health Study." *Child Abuse and Neglect* 25 (4): 557–84.

Penn, William. 1998. *As We Are Now: Mixblood Essays on Race and Identity*. Los Angeles: University of California Press.

Perdue, Theda. 2003. *"Mixed Blood" Indians: Racial Construction in the Early South*. Athens: University of Georgia Press.

Pevar, Stephen L. 1992. *The Rights of Indians and Tribes*. Carbondale: Southern Illinois University Press.

Poston, Walker. 1990. "The Biracial Identity Development Model: A Needed Addition." *Journal of Counseling and Development* 69 (2): 152–55.

Purcell, David, Lisa Metsch, Mary Latka, Cynthia Gomez, Carl Latkin, Yuko Mizuno, and the IN-

SPIRE Team. 2004. "Behavioral Prevention Trial with HIV-Seropositive Injection Drug Users: Rationale and Methods of the INSPIRE Study." *Journal of Acquired Immune Deficiency Syndrome* 37 (Supplement 2): S110–18.

Purcell, David, Lisa Metsch, Mary Latka, Scott Santibanez, Cynthia Gomez, Lois Eldred, and Carl Latkin. 2007. "Results from a Randomized Controlled Trial of a Peer-Mentoring Intervention to Reduce HIV Transmission and Increase Access to Care and Adherence to HIV Medications among HIV-Seropositive Injection Drug Users." *Journal of Acquired Immune Deficiency Syndrome* 46 (Supplement 2): S37–45.

Ramirez, Renya. 2007. *Native Hubs: Culture, Community, and Belonging in Silicon Valley and Beyond.* Durham, NC: Duke University Press.

Renn, Kristen. 2000. "Patterns of Situational Identity among Biracial and Multiracial College Students." *Review of Higher Education* 23 (4): 399–420.

———. 2003. "Understanding the Identities of Mixed-Race College Students through a Developmental Ecology Lens." *Journal of College Student Development* 44 (3): 383–403.

———. 2004. *Mixed Race Students in College: The Ecology of Race, Identity, and Community.* Albany: SUNY Press.

———. 2008. "Research on Biracial and Multiracial Identity Development: Overview and Synthesis." In *Biracial and Multiracial Students: New Directions for Student Services,* Special Edition, no. 123, edited by Kristen Renn and Paul Shang, 13–21. New York: Jossey-Bass.

Robert Wood Johnson Foundation. 2007. *Invisible Tribes: Urban Indians and Their Health in a Changing World.* www.rwjf.org/en/about-rwjf/newsroom/newsroom-content/2007/11/significant-health-care-needs-of-american-indians-and-alaska-nat.html. Accessed October 25, 2013.

Root, Maria. 1990. "Resolving 'Other' Status: Identity Development of Biracial Individuals." *Women and Therapy* 9 (1–2): 185–205.

———. 1992. *Racially Mixed People in America.* Thousand Oaks, CA: Sage Publications.

———. 1995. *The Multiracial Experience: Racial Borders as the Next Frontier.* Thousand Oaks, CA: Sage Publications.

———. 1998. "Experiences and Processes Affecting Racial Identity Development: Preliminary Results from the Biracial Sibling Project." *Cultural Diversity and Mental Health* 4 (3): 237–47.

———. 2003. "Racial Identity Development and Persons of Mixed Race Heritage." In *Multiracial Child Resource Book: Living Complex Identities,* edited by Maria Root and Matthew Kelley, 34–41. Seattle: MAVIN Foundation.

Roscoe, Will. 1988. *Living the Spirit: A Gay American Indian Anthology.* New York: St. Martin's Griffin.

———. 2000 (1988). *Changing Ones: Third and Fourth Genders in Native North America,* New York: Palgrave Macmillan.

Sandoval, Chela. 2000. *Methodology of the Oppressed.* Minneapolis: University of Minnesota Press.

Saunt, Claudio. 2005. *Black, White, and Indian: Race and the Unmaking of an American Family.* New York: Oxford University Press.

Simpson, Audra. 2014. *Mohawk Interruptus: Political Life across the Borders of Settler States.* Durham, NC: Duke University Press.

Simpson, Leanne. 2013. *Islands of Decolonial Love.* Winnipeg: Arbeiter Ring Publishing.

Singer, Beverly. 2001. *Wiping the Warpaint Off the Lens: Native American Film and Video.* Minneapolis: University of Minnesota Press.

Smith, Andrea. 1999. "Sexual Violence and American Indian Genocide." In *Remembering Conquest: Feminist/Womanist Perspectives on Religion, Colonization and Sexual Violence,* edited by Nantawan Boonprasat Lewis and Marie M. Fortune, 31–52. Binghamton, NY: Haworth Press.

Smith, Linda Tuhiwai. 1999. *Decolonizing Methodologies: Research and Indigenous Peoples.* London: Zed Books.

Solomon, Julie, Jacqueline Berman, and Josefina Card. 2007. *Tools for Building Culturally Competent HIV Prevention Programs*. New York: Spring Publishing.

Spickard, Paul. 1991. *Mixed-Blood: Intermarriage and Ethnic Identity in Twentieth Century America*. Madison: University of Wisconsin Press.

Stall, Ron, Thomas Mills, John Williamson, Trevor Hart, Greg Greenwood, Jay Paul, Lance Pollack, et al. 2003. "Association of Co-Occurring Psychosocial Health Problems and Increased Vulnerability to HIV/AIDS among Urban Men Who Have Sex with Men." *American Journal of Public Health* 93 (6): 939–42.

Stonequist, Everett. 1937. *The Marginal Man: A Study in Personality and Culture Conflict*. New York: Charles Scribner's Sons.

Sturm, Circe. 2002. *Blood Politics: Race, Culture, and Identity in the Cherokee Nation of Oklahoma*. Berkeley: University of California Press.

Sue, Derald, Christina Capodilupo, Gina Torino, Jennifer Bucceri, Aisha Holder, Kevin Nadal, and Marta Esquilin. 2007. "Racial Microaggressions in Everyday Life: Implications for Clinical Practice." *American Journal of Psychology* 62 (4): 271–86.

Tashiro, Cathy. 2005. "Health Disparities in the Context of Mixed Race Challenging the Ideology of Race." *Advances in Nursing Science* 28 (3): 203–11.

Tinker, George. 1993. *Missionary Conquest: The Gospel and Native American Cultural Genocide*. Minneapolis: Fortress Press.

United Nations, with the Native American Solidarity Committee. 1977. *The Systematic Genocide of Native Nations by the United States Government*. Published as a monograph by the American Indian Treaty Council. San Francisco: Freedom Archives.

Urban Indian Health Commission. 2007. *Invisible Tribes: Urban Indians and Their Health in a Changing World*. www.uihi.org/download/UIHC_Report_FINAL.pdf. Accessed October 25, 2013.

U.S. Census Bureau. 2000, 2012, 2014. U.S. Census. www.census.gov. Accessed October 28, 2013.

Valleroy, Linda, Duncan MacKellar, John Karon, Daniel Rosen, William McFarland, Douglas Shehan, and Susan Stoyanoff. 2000. "HIV Prevalence and Associated Risks in Young Men Who Have Sex with Men." *Journal of the American Medical Association* 284 (2): 198–204.

Vernaci, Lorenzo. 2010. *Settler Colonialism: A Theoretical Overview*. New York: Palgrave Macmillan.

Vernon, Irene. 2001. *Killing Us Quietly: Native Americans and HIV/AIDS*. Lincoln, NE: Bison Books.

Vestal, Christine. 2013. "Affordable Care Act a Hard Sell for Native Americans." *USA Today*, October 15, 2013.

Walters, Karina, and Jane Simoni. 2002. "Re-Cnceptualizing Native Women's Health: An 'Indigenist' Stress-Coping Model." *American Journal of Public Health* 92 (4): 520–24.

Walters, Karina, Jane Simoni, and Tessa Evans-Campbell. 2002. "Substance Use among American Indians and Alaska Natives: Incorporating Culture in an 'Indigenist' Stress-Coping Paradigm." *Public Health Reports* 117 (Supplement 1): S104–17.

Walters, Karina, Tessa Evans-Campbell, Jane Simoni, Theresa Ronquillo, and Rupaleem Bhuyan. 2006. "'My Spirit Is in My Heart': Identity Experiences and Challenges among American Indian Two-Spirit Women." *Journal of Lesbian Studies* 10 (1–2): 125–49.

Walters, Karina, Tessa Evans-Campbell, Ramona Beltran, and Jane Simoni. 2011. "Keeping Our Hearts from Touching the Ground: HIV/AIDS in American Indian and Alaska Native Women." *Journal of Women's Health Issues* 21 (6 Suppl): S261–65.

Warrior, Robert Allen. 1995. *Tribal Secrets: Recovering American Indian Intellectual Traditions*. Minneapolis: University of Minnesota Press.

Waters, Mary. 2000. "Immigration, Intermarriage, and the Challenges of Measuring Racial/Ethnic Identities." *American Journal of Public Health* 90 (11): 1735–37.

Wijeyesinghe, Charmaine. 2001. "Racial Identity in Multiracial People: An Alternative Paradigm." In *New Perspectives on Racial Identity Development: A Theoretical and Practical Anthology*, edited by Charmaine Wijeyesinghe and Bailey Jackson III, 129–52. New York: New York University Press.

Wijeyesinghe, Charmaine, and Bailey Jackson. 2012. *New Perspectives on Racial Identity Development: Integrating Emerging Frameworks*. New York: New York University Press.

Wilson, Kathleen. 2003. "Therapeutic Landscapes and First Nations Peoples: An Exploration of Culture, Health and Place." *Health and Place* 9 (2): 83–93.

Wilson, Shawn. 2009. *Research Is Ceremony: Indigenous Research Methods*. Halifax, NS: Fernwood Publishing.

Wilson, Terry. 1993. "Blood Quantum: Native American Mixed Bloods." In *Racially Mixed People in America*, edited by Maria Root, 108–25. Thousand Oaks, CA: Sage Publications.

Wilson, Waziyatawin Angela, and Michael Yellow Bird. 2005. *For Indigenous Eyes Only: A Decolonization Handbook*. Santa Fe: School of American Research Press.

Wilson, William Julius. 1980. *The Declining Significance of Race: Blacks and Changing American Institutions*. Chicago: University of Chicago Press.

Yellow Horse Brave Heart, Maria. 2003. "The Historical Trauma Response among Natives and Its Relationship with Substance Abuse: A Lakota Illustration." *Journal of Psychoactive Drugs* 35 (1): 108–25.

YWCA. "Violence against Women Act (VAWA)." www.ywca.org/site/c.cuIRJ7NTKrLaG/b.8864563/k.319C/Violence_Against_Women_Act_VAWA.htm. Accessed November 10, 2013.

Zimmerman, Marc. 1995. "Psychological Empowerment: Issues and Illustrations." *American Journal of Community Psychology* 23 (5): 581–99.

INDEX

aboriginal science, 49

Affordable Care Act, 7, 52, 113, 127

AIM (American Indian Movement), 43

Alarcon, Norma, 141n2

American Indian and Alaska Natives of
mixed descent (AIANs), 46, 142n3

American Indian studies, xi, 5, 81

ancestor spirits, 29, 91, 102–7

Anishinaabe, 16

anthropological power, 17

anthropological studies, 17

anti-miscegenation, 40, 80

Apache, 16

Arapahoe, 16

ascription model, 20, 29, 63, 98

Asian Pacific Islander (API) Wellness Center, 114–15

authenticity, 12, 19–21, 35, 38–40, 69, 77, 80, 107, 110, 130, 133

bad blood, 12

Barker, Joanne, 39, 69–70

Bay Area American Indian Two-Spirits
(BAAITS), 20, 42, 57, 83, 111, 113–15, 117, 132, 135–37

Benoit, Joan, 14

berdache identity, 17, 35

bisexual, 9, 14–15, 20, 24, 32, 65, 91–92

Black community, 23, 25, 71, 76, 80–81, 143n3 (chap. 4)

Blackfeet, 16

blood, 5–10, 12–14, 16, 18–21, 23, 25–26, 28–30, 31–33, 35, 38–40, 43, 45, 49, 50, 55, 56, 60–64, 70–74, 77–79, 86, 94, 95, 107, 108–13, 122, 126, 128–30, 135, 138–39, 143n1 (chap. 5), 143n2 (chap. 5). *See also* mixed-blood

blood quantum, 13, 18–20, 38, 73, 74, 78, 86, 128–30

Bonilla-Silva, Eduardo, 71, 79

boté, 33–34

building blocks of cultural competence, 117

Burns, Gayle, 14

Canadian AIDS Society, 144n3

Cass Model, 13, 141n3

Centers for Disease Control (CDC), 7, 24, 46, 142n3

ceremonial healing, 9, 32

ceremonial return, 28

Certificate of Degree of Indian Blood
(CDIB), 20

Cheng, Patrick, xi, 5

Cherokee, 10–11, 13, 16, 20, 39, 76, 78, 88, 124, 130–31

Chickasaw, 16

Chippewa, 16

Choctaw, 16

circle, 14, 56, 87, 103, 112, 135, 137

class, 16, 25, 67, 69, 71, 142n2 (chap. 4)

cognitive dissonance, mixed-race, 9, 28–29, 32–33, 43–44, 59, 74, 76–90, 91, 96, 100, 121

Cohen, Cathy, 25–26, 143n3 (chap. 4)

colonial haunting, 6, 12, 17–18, 20, 26, 27, 30, 33, 46, 49, 50, 54–55, 58, 63, 72, 77, 80, 85, 93, 102, 107, 118, 122, 137–39

colonial trauma, x, 12, 29, 49, 116, 118–19, 124, 136, 138

colonization, 6, 10, 12, 32, 36, 46, 51, 52, 62, 77, 80, 81, 93, 104, 107, 111, 122, 136, 142n1 (chap. 2)

colorblind theories, 71, 143n2 (chap. 4)

colorism, 118, 119

communal healing, 122, 137–39

consensus issues, 25–26

Cook-Lynn, Elizabeth, 62

Cornell, Stephen, 73

Cree, 6, 16, 141n1 (chap. 1)

Creek, 6

indigenous cosmologies, 37
Indigenous cultural mentoring networks
     (ICMNs), 124, 128, 130
Indigenous knowledge, 5, 59, 73, 136
Indigenous methodologies, 6
Indigenous studies, x, xi, 19, 73, 80
Indigenous Wellness Research Institute,
     University of Washington, xiv, 5
intergenerational healing and cultural lead-
     ership intervention model (IHCL), 28,
     45, 134, 136, 137–8
intergenerational love, 138–39
intergenerational mentoring, 9, 32, 136
intergenerational trauma, 56–59, 65, 67, 77,
     81, 84–86, 90, 91, 92, 95, 97, 106, 121,
     125, 134–36. *See also* trauma
internalized oppression, 29, 40, 67, 106
intersectionality, 69

Kaiser, 118, 127, 129
Kawerak, 16
kinship, ix, 13, 30, 54, 62, 72, 74, 83, 90, 105,
     106, 113, 115, 136
kinship networks, 9, 28, 32, 34, 41, 44, 45,
     81, 83, 109, 110, 112, 113, 116, 122, 125,
     134, 135
Klopotek, Brian, 80, 81, 111

Lakota, 16, 106, 130, 131
LGBTQ, 6, 13, 14, 16, 34, 50, 60, 61, 72, 92,
     95, 132, 133
Lopez, Andru, 14
Lyons, Scott Richard, 72

Mandan, 16
Mannheim, Karl, 144n2
Medicare, 113, 127
Mellers, Barbara, 96
men who have sex with men (MSM), 20, 23,
     25, 26, 94
Mestizo, 16
Micmac, 16
microaggressions, 63
mixed-blood, 6, 9, 13, 14, 16, 29, 43, 45, 56,
     61, 62, 72, 77, 107, 108, 112, 126, 135, 138,
     143n1 (chap. 5), 143n2 (chap. 5). *See
     also* blood
mixed-heritage, 34
mixed-race cognitive dissonance, 9, 28, 43,

44, 74, 81, 84, 86, 88, 90, 91, 96, 100, 121
mixed-race identity, 4, 7–10, 14, 19, 26, 27,
     37, 40, 41, 50, 72, 81, 84, 107, 116, 118,
     122, 131, 137, 139
mixed-race metronomic subject, 76, 78
mixed-race, queer-identified, transgender,
     and/or Two-Spirit (MLGBTQ2S), xii, 9,
     12, 13, 16–17, 19–23, 25–30, 32, 34–39, 41,
     42, 45–50, 54–59, 60–68, 70–78, 80–90,
     91–97, 100, 102–07, 110–20, 122–38,
     141n3
mixed-race studies, xi, xiv, 8, 76, 82
monoracial, 25, 29, 41, 82, 87
Morgensen, Scott, 16, 17, 21, 32, 35, 38, 39
multiracial identification, 76
multiracial identity, 80, 81, 82, 87, 110
Muñoz, José, 61, 62, 63, 98, 142n1 (chap. 4)

National Alliance of State and Territorial
     AIDS Directors (NASTAD), 54
National Coalition of Anti-Violence Pro-
     grams, 92, 143n2 (chap. 6)
nationalism, 13, 62, 72
nation-people, 72, 73
Native American AIDS Project (NAAP),
     xiii, 14, 15, 22, 23, 31, 41, 42, 49, 55–59,
     64, 83, 85, 86, 99, 102, 111, 114–19, 122,
     134, 137
Native American Health Center (NAHC),
     86, 110, 111, 114, 115, 117, 134, 136, 137
Native hubs, 111
Native-specific organizations, 35, 111, 112,
     115, 116, 118, 127, 128
Native studies, x, 18, 92
Navajo Nation, 4, 39
Naya Ji, 16
neoliberalism, 71, 143n2 (chap. 4)
normativity, 38

Obama, Barack, 7, 71, 92, 113
Office of Federal Acknowledgement, 69
Ohlone, 16
Ojibwa, 16
Osage, 16, 74

Paiute, 16, 103
pan-Indian, 11, 83, 128, 130
peer-mentoring programs, 125
peyote, 104–05

talking circle, 14
Tepetuan, 16
third gender, 32, 33
third-generation return, 109
traditional urban Indian cultural knowledge
 systems (TUICKS), 30, 110–12, 122, 124,
 125, 130, 131, 133, 134, 136–37
transgender, ix, x, xii, 9, 14–15, 20, 24, 31,
 32, 34, 35, 45, 56, 60, 64, 65, 67, 87, 88,
 91, 93, 98, 99, 100, 101, 115, 116, 120, 121,
 141n1 (chap. 2), 143n5
trauma, ix, x, xii, 6, 9, 10, 12, 13, 26–29, 32,
 33, 37, 42, 44–45, 47–59, 65, 91, 95, 96,
 97, 100, 101, 102, 109, 116, 118–19, 123,
 124, 125, 134–35, 136, 138, 139, 142n2
 (chap. 2), 144n2, 144n3. *See also* intergenerational trauma
tribal affiliation, 16
tribal sovereignty, 18, 21, 62, 74
triple marginalization, 26, 29
Two-Spirit, ix–xii, 6, 9–16, 17–22, 24, 27–28,
 29–30, 32–38, 41–43, 45–47, 50, 59–61,
 66–67, 72, 81, 86, 90, 91, 95, 103, 105,
 107, 118, 121, 122, 124–25, 132–36, 139,
 141n2 (chap. 1), 142n2 (chap. 2)
Two-Spirit cultural dissolution, 9, 12, 28, 29,
 32–39, 42, 43, 45, 46, 59, 67, 81, 86, 90,
 91, 105, 118, 121, 135
Two-Spirit cultural ethic of reciprocity, 32
Two-Spirit Powwow, x

U.N. Declaration on the Rights of Indigenous Peoples, 54
United Nations, 54, 143n3 (chap. 5)
urban environments, 27, 102, 109
urban Indian kinship networks, 9, 28, 29,
 32, 45, 81, 83, 108, 110, 112, 113, 116, 122,
 125, 135, 144
U.S. Census, 8, 40, 41
U.S. government, 8, 20, 38, 40, 51, 53, 73,
 108, 127, 143n3 (chap. 5)

Valleroy, Linda, 23, 25, 26
Vernon, Irene, 37
Violence against Women Act (VAWA), 92,
 143n1 (chap. 6)
vulnerability, 5, 47, 49, 56, 59, 68, 92, 95,
 96, 97

Wabanaki, 16
Walters, Karina, 5, 37, 46, 55, 63, 69, 111,
 144n3
Warrior, Robert, 74
Western science, 49–50
Wilson, Shawn, 6, 141n1 (chap. 1)
Wilson, William Julius, 71, 142n2 (chap. 4)

Zuni, 141n1 (chap. 2)

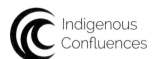 Indigenous
Confluences

Charlotte Cotè, Matthew Sakiestewa Gilbert,
and Coll Thrush, *Series Editors*

Indigenous Confluences publishes innovative works that use decolonizing perspectives and transnational approaches to explore the experiences of Indigenous peoples across North America, with special emphasis on the Pacific Coast.